A NEWLY DISCOVERED SYSTEM

OF

ELECTRICAL MEDICATION.

By DANIEL CLARK, A.M.

CINCINNATI:
PRINTED BY HITCHCOCK AND WALDEN,
FOR THE AUTHOR.
1875.

PREFACE.

In the summer of 1866, the author of this little book, moved by the repeated and earnest solicitation of his Medical Classes, prepared and printed a small pamphlet entitled *Practical Principles of Medical Electricity*, designed more particularly, as the present work also is, as a *Hand-Book* to assist the memory of those who have taken a regular course of Lectures from himself, or from some other competent instructor in the same general system of Practice. The edition of that work was exhausted somewhat more than a year ago. Still, the book has continued to be frequently called for. The author has, therefore, prepared, and now offers to the Profession, the present volume, comprising the substance of the previous work—corrected, improved in arrangement and form, and about doubled in size by the introduction of new matter. While he has reason for gratitude that the former manual, referred to above, has met with so favorable a reception, he can not but hope that the present work will be found even more acceptable and valuable to both practitioners and their patients.

It is but justice to say that the most essential principles of *practice* here presented did not originate with the present author, but with PROF. C. H. BOLLES, of Philadelphia, their discoverer, from whom the writer received his first introduction to them. Yet, the *explanations* here given of the Law of Polarization, as respects the electric current in the circuit of the artificial machine, as well as respecting the natural magnets and magnetic currents of the human organism; the introduction of the *long cord*, with the explanation of its advantages; and also nearly everything of the *philosophic theories* here brought to view, the author alone is responsible for.

This work, like its little predecessor from the same pen, has been adapted exclusively to the use of DR. JEROME KIDDER'S Electro-Magnetic Machine, manufactured and sold, at present, at No. 544 Broadway, New York; because the author, having used in his own practice a considerable variety of the most popular machines intended for therapeutic purposes, and having examined several others, believes this to be incomparably *the best in use.* Dr. Kidder has, with most laudable zeal, pressed on his researches and improvements in the manufacture of these instruments, until there seems to be scarcely anything more in them to be desired. They are certainly not equalled by any others in America, and probably not surpassed, if equalled, by any in the world.

D. C.

Plainfield, Ill., June, 1869.

CONTENTS.

PRINCIPLES OF PRACTICE.

PRESCRIPTIONS.

INTRODUCTION.

Considerable parts of this book have been written for the unlearned. For the scholarly reader such parts, of course, would be wholly superfluous; yet it is hoped that they to whom these are familiar will be patient in passing through them for the sake of others to whom they may be instructive. Other parts, again, it is believed, will be found new to the most of even educated minds. But men of the largest intellectual attainments are commonly the most docile. Such men, meeting this little work, will not shrink from a candid examination of its contents merely on account of their comparative novelty, nor because the views expressed differ essentially from those usually held by the medical faculty. The candid, yet critical, attention of such gentlemen, the author especially solicits. He assures them that he does not write at random, but from careful research and practical experience. His *philosophic theories* he offers only for what they are worth. His *principles of practice* he believes to be scientifically correct and of great value.

Let it not be supposed that the author, in this work, assumes a belligerent attitude towards the members of the medical profession. Although anxious to modify and elevate their estimate of electricity as a remedial agent, and to improve their methods of using it, he has no sympathy with those who profess to believe, and who assert, that medicines of the apothecary never effect the cure of disease; that where they are thought to cure, they simply do not kill; and who contend that the patient would have recovered quicker and better to have taken no medicine at all. He knows that such allegations are false, as they are extravagant; and so does every candid and unprejudiced observer whose experience has given him ordinary opportunities to judge. The writer believes it can be perfectly demonstrated that the advancement of medical science in modern times—say within the last two or three hundred years—has served to essentially prolong the average term of human life. The world owes to medical instructors and practitioners a debt of gratitude which can never be paid. Their laborious and often perilous research in the fields of their profession, and their untiring assiduity in the application of their science and skill to the relief of human suffering, entitle them to a degree of confidence and affectionate esteem which few other classes of public servants can rightly claim. For one, the author of this little book most sincerely concedes to them, as a body, his confidence, his sympathy, and his grateful respect. And the most that he is willing to say to their discredit, (if it be so construed), is that he regards them as having not yet attained *perfection* in their high profession, and as not being generally as willing as they should be to examine fairly into the alleged merits of remedial agents and improved principles of practice, (claimed to be such), when brought forward by intelligent, cultivated and respectable men, outside of "the regular profession." This is said at the same time that the author gives much weight to their commonly offered defense, viz: that, in the midst of professional engagements, they have not always the time to spare for such examination; and that, since the most of alleged improvements in the healing art, particularly of those introduced by persons who have not received a regular medical education, sooner or later prove themselves to be worthless, the *presumption*—though not the *certainty*—is, whenever a new agent, or a new method or principle is proposed by an "outsider," that this, too, if not willful charlatanism, is a mistake; and therefore, the sooner it comes to an end the better it will be for the public health, and that neglect is the surest way to kill it.

But the medical faculty have too widely employed electricity in the treatment of disease, and that with too frequent success, to admit of its being denied a place among important therapeutic agents by any respectable practitioner. The only questions concerning it now are those which relate to the *versatility* of its power, the *scope* of its useful applicability, and the *principles* which should guide in the administration of it. The general subject embraced in these questions is one in which suffering humanity has a right to claim that physicians shall be at home.

And yet it will scarcely be denied that, in the exhibition of electricity, more than of almost any other therapeutic agent, medical practitioners feel incertitude as to what shall be its effect. Now and then it acts as they expected it to do; sometimes it pleasantly surprises them; oftener it offensively disappoints them. They find it *unreliable.* Of other remedial agents, they commonly know, before administering them, what *sort* of effect will be produced; but in employing this, while they have hope, they are generally more or less in doubt. They regard it as *a stimulant;* although its action on the living organism appears to them to be largely veiled in mystery. In many cases of disease, particularly those of acutely inflammatory or febrile character, they judge it to be not at all indicated. To administer it in a case of bilious or typhoid fever, or in a case of pneumonia, pleuritis, gastritis, inflammatory rheumatism, or acute, and especially *epidemic* or malignant dysentery, or in a case of pulmonary phthisis, would probably be viewed by the most of physicians as the rashest empiricism, if not the next thing to madness. *The idea of producing antagonistic effects with it at will,* they would, for the most part, esteem preposterous. Rather, perhaps, it may be said of the majority of medical practitioners that such an idea has never entered their minds; so foreign is it to their conceptions of truth and propriety. But, at whatever risk of discredit or censure, the writer of the present volume avers that this idea is both scientifically sound and of every day's practical verification. The various and opposite forms of disease—acute and chronic, hypersthenic and asthenic—are habitually treated and *cured*, in his own practice and that of his students, by electricity alone.

But "*cui bono?*" may be asked. "What if it be true that these things can be done with electricity? They are also done with medicines, which are more quickly and conveniently administered, and usually less annoying to the patient. What, therefore, is the *practical utility* of your electric system above the ordinary practice, especially if we include, in the latter, electrical treatment as occasionally employed by the most of respectable physicians?"

This is the important question—that to which the author desires to call particular attention. He, therefore, answers:

First.—It is manifestly true that the most of diseases, (the exceptions are comparatively few), can be cured by the use of medicines. It is also true that these can generally be administered with more convenience and less expenditure of time to the practitioner than electricity; and this is a great advantage. The author is often asked if he thinks his electric system will ever supersede the use of medicines. His answer is uniformly, "No." It takes too much time for that. Where the population is crowded, as in cities and large towns, it is often the case, especially in times of prevailing epidemic, that a physician can prescribe medicine for half a dozen or more patients in the time required to treat one electrically. To reject medicines and rely alone on electricity would, in periods and places of prevailing sickness, leave many sufferers without professional service, or would require that the proportion of doctors to the whole population should be largely increased—a thing certainly not often to be desired. So much, candor must concede.

Second.—It is not quite true that medicines are usually less annoying to the patient than electricity as *we* use it. As administered by others, it is often nearly intolerable. In our hands, on the contrary, it seldom inflicts any pain or distress, and almost invariably becomes agreeable to the patient after a very few applications. We have no occasion to torture our patients in order to cure them. But the cases are comparatively rare where medicines are not offensive; commonly they are excessively so.

Third.—In not a few diseases, and these among the most dangerous or distressful, the electric current, employed according to the system here taught, is able to reach, control and cure, with facility, where medicines are but slowly, and in most instances imperfectly successful, or fail altogether. This is said, or meant to be said, not invidiously nor boastingly, but in the candid utterance of a great and practically demonstrated truth. It is, perhaps, most *often* exemplified in neuralgic, rheumatic and paralytic affections. The author is happy to acknowledge that these diseases are frequently mitigated, and occasionally cured, by means of electrical treatment administered by those who know nothing of the system here taught. But the important fact is, in *their* hands there is *no certainty* as to the effect before trial. Under *this* system, the kind of effect is as certainly known before as after the trial, since it can be made one thing or another *at will.*

Cases are not unfrequently presented of *inflammatory action*, more especially where it is internal—traumatic cases and others—which the practitioner finds it impossible to subdue with medicine. But, with a proper knowledge of the system herein taught, he has at his command a power with which he can control such cases with almost infallible certainty, provided he can get access to them within reasonable time. The same may be said of fevers, particularly those occasioned by miasmatic or infectious virus. These are often difficult to manage by the use of medicine, and not seldom prove fatal, in spite of the best talent and skill which the profession can afford. But the electric current, rightly selected and scientifically applied, destroys or neutralizes the virus and restores the normal polarization, and so effects a cure.

Neuralgic affections are frequently found difficult, or even impossible, to be cured by means of medicines, and yet, in the very same cases, these affections yield and disappear with comparative facility when brought under the electric current, judiciously applied, according to the principles of this new system,

Chronic cases, and others of an asthenic character, are often very stubborn under the medicines of pharmacy, and are commonly the dread of physicians; yet, under scientific treatment by electricity, they rarely fail to lose their formidable character and to become obedient to the remedial agent.

Fourth.—In enumerating a few of the peculiar advantages of this system, I should add that it corrects the usual *electric* practice of the profession, so far as they become acquainted with it. As before intimated, the mass of physicians at present, who treat more or less electrically, do so with no knowledge, or next to none, of the great *versatility* of action of which the electric current is capable. They know nothing of the electrical polarization of the living organism in health, nor how it is variously affected in disease. The particular *electrical* state of the diseased organs is a matter foreign to their minds. They appear to suppose the point to be immediately aimed at as a means of cure is to get the electricity from the machine into the affected part or parts; whereas it should be to change, by correction, the *polarization* of the part or parts; and, if there be virus present, to neutralize that. Equally unacquainted are they generally with the diverse physiological action of the several modifications of the electric force—galvanism, magnetism, faradaism, and frictional electricity. This, in their candor, they commonly acknowledge. And, for the most part, they are little or nothing better acquainted with the *distinctive* effects on the system of the positive and negative poles of the instrument. There is, therefore, plainly no *science* in their electrical practice. Every thing is done at random—all is empirical.

But the system here taught opens the light upon all of these points. For practical purposes, at least, it is, in its essential features, the only system of electrical therapeutics which has in it any real merit—the only system which *can be true.* By this, the writer does not mean to assert, or to imply, that the little book now before the reader contains no error, either in respect to theory or practice. In this early stage of our system's history, it would be remarkable if it did not contain errors in both these respects. But what it is intended to affirm is, that the book presents the *cardinal features* of a true, and the only possibly true, system of electrical practice. All possibly true systems of geometry must necessarily be essentially the same; and so, too, all possibly true systems of electrical medication must be essentially one. That one system, it is candidly and confidently believed, is briefly contained in the present little volume.

ELECTRICAL MEDICATION.

FIRST PRINCIPLES.

DR. JEROME KIDDER'S ELECTRO-MAGNETIC MACHINE.

ON opening the machine-box, as it comes from the manufacturer, there will be found a glass bottle, intended to hold the battery fluid when not in use; a glass cup or jar, to serve as the battery cell; a pair of insulated metallic conducting cords; two tin electrodes; a brass clamp; and, under the helix-box, (which raise), the battery metals and two connecting wires to unite the battery with the helix.

To put the machine in working condition—ready for use—proceed, step by step, as follows, viz: Prepare the *Battery Fluid* by mixing twelve parts, by measure, of water with one part of sulphuric acid, (good commercial acid is pure enough), sufficient to fill the cell two-thirds or three-fourths full, and place in it about one-third of an ounce of quicksilver.

Next, place the platina plate between the two zinc plates, standing on their legs upon a table before you; and bring the top of the wooden bar (in a groove of which the platina is set) up flush with the top of the zinc plates. Let the brass post, standing on the top of this bar and soldered to the platina plate below, be toward the left-hand side. Then take the brass clamp and place it across the top of these metallic plates, a little to the right of the brass post, or about midway between the right and left sides, having its thumb-screw towards you, and with it screw the three plates firmly together. The platina is shorter than the zincs, to prevent its reaching the quicksilver in the bottom of the cell; and the wax balls on its sides are to insulate it from the zinc plates. This platina should never be allowed to touch the mercury or the zinc.

Let the plates, properly screwed together, be now placed in the cell with the Battery Fluid. Then, with the two copper connecting-wires, connect the post which stands on the wooden bar above the platina with the post stamped P on the helix-box, and the brass clamp N with the post N on the helix-box.

If, now, the screws regulating the vibrating armature be in perfect adjustment, the current will commence to run, with a buzzing sound; or it may be made to start by touching the hammer-like head of the flat steel spring. If not, the screws may be rightly adjusted in the following way: The top screw, which at its lower point is tipped with a small coil of platina wire, should be made to press delicately upon the center of the little iron plate on the upper side of the spring, so as to bear the latter down very slightly. Then raise or depress the screw-magnet, which turns up or down under the hammer, like the seat of a piano-stool, until the vibration of the spring commences. The *rapidity of the vibrations*, by which is secured the alternate closing and breaking of the electric circuit (or rather what, in practical effect, is equivalent to this—the *direct* and *reverse* action of the current in alternation) is increased by raising the screw-magnet and diminished by lowering it. When it is raised above what is required for ordinary use, the noise becomes too loud and harsh for many nervous patients to bear. It should then be depressed a little.

With respect to curative power, I have discovered but little perceptible difference, produced by the various degrees of rapidity in the vibrations, effected within the range of this magnet.

The force of the current is regulated by means of a tubular magnet, which slides over the helix, and is called *the plunger*. It is approached under a brass cap at the right-hand end of the machine. The plunger is withdrawn, more or less, to increase the force; pushed in to diminish it. If in any case the current can not be softened sufficiently with the plunger, the quantity of battery fluid in use must be made less.

After a time the current will become weak, and fail to run well. Then renew the battery fluid. When the quicksilver is all taken up by the zinc plates, the machine may be run for a while without adding more. But after it has considerably disappeared from the inside surface of the zinc plates, the latter will begin to show more rapid corrosion, while the current will be less. Then let a small quantity of quicksilver—one-fourth to one-third of an ounce—again be placed in the fluid.

When the machine is not in use, let the metals be removed from the fluid; and, if not to be soon again used, let them be rinsed with water, carefully avoiding to wet the wooden bar in which the platina is set.

The posts, with which the conducting-cords are to be connected, are arranged in a row near the front of the helix-box, and are marked A, B, C, D. Either two of these posts may be used to obtain a current; and since they admit of six varying combinations, six different currents are afforded by the machine, viz: the A B current, the A C current, the A D current, the B C current, the B D current, and the C D current. Whichever current is used, it may always be known which of the two posts employed is the positive and which the negative, by observing the letters stamped upon their tops. The one whose letter comes first in the order of the alphabet is positive; the other is negative. Also, the one standing towards the left hand is positive, and that at the right hand is negative. *The qualities* of the several currents are stated in a descriptive paper on the inside of the lid of the machine, which see. It will there be found that three of the currents—viz, the A B, the A C and the A D currents—are *electrolytic:* that is, dissolving by electric action. These electrolytic currents require to be used—one or another of them—whenever any chemical action is needed; as, in decomposing or neutralizing *virus* in the system, destroying cancers, reducing glands when chronically enlarged, removing tumors or other abnormal growths, and in treating old ulcers and chronic irritation of mucous membranes. The other three, being Faradaic or induction currents, and having no perceptibly chemical action, are used where only change of electro-vital polarization is required. These Faradaic currents differ from each other in respect to being *concentrative* or *diffusive* in their effects, and in their *sensational* force. B C is concentrative and delicately sensational. C D is also concentrative, though less so than B C, and is more strongly sensational. B D is diffusive, and the most energetically sensational of the three.

POLARIZATION.

It may be proper, in this place, to spend a few words upon electrical polarization in general.

Electrical polarity may be defined as a characteristic of the electric or magnetic fluid, by virtue of which its opposite qualities, as those of *attraction* and *repulsion* towards the same object, are manifested in opposite parts of the electric or magnetic body. These opposite parts are called the *poles* of the body, as the *positive* and *negative* poles. The difference between the positive and negative poles is believed to be that of *plus* and *minus*—plus being positive and minus negative. This is the Franklinian view, and, if I mistake not, is the one most in favor with men of science at the present day. This view supposes that the electricity or magnetism arranges itself in *maximum* quantity and intensity at the one extremity or pole of the magnetized body, and in *minimum* quantity and intensity at the opposite extremity or pole; and that, between these points—the maximum and the minimum—the fluid is distributed, in respect to quantity and intensity, upon a scale of regular graduation from the one to the other. The idea may be represented by a *line*, commencing in a *point* at the one end, and extending, with regularly increasing breadth, to the other end. The larger end would represent the positive pole, and the smaller, the negative pole. Or perhaps a better representation of the magnet would be a line of equal breadth from end to end, but having the one end *white*, or slightly tinted, say, with *red*, and the color gradually and regularly increasing in strength to the other end, where it becomes a *deep scarlet*. Let the coloring-matter represent the magnetism in the body charged, and we have the magnet illustrated in its polarization: the deep-red end is the positive pole, and the white or faintly-colored end is the negative pole.

It is a law of polarization that the positive poles of different magnets repel each other, and the negative poles repel each other; while positive and negative poles attract each other. The same law of polarization rules in electric or magnetic *currents* as in magnets at rest.

THE ELECTRIC CIRCUIT.

The Electric Circuit is made up of any thing and every thing which serves to conduct the electric current in its passage—outward and returning—from where it leaves the inner surfaces of the zinc plates in the battery cell to where it comes back again to the outer surfaces of the same plates. When the conducting-cords are not attached to the machine, or when the communication between the cords is not complete, if the machine be running, the circuit is then composed of the battery fluid, the platina plate, the posts, the connecting-wires, which unite the battery with the helix, the helical wires, and their appendages for the vibrating action. But when a patient is under treatment, the conducting-cords, the electrodes, and so much of the patient's person as is traversed by the current while passing from the positive electrode through to the negative electrode, are also included in the whole circuit. And whatever elements may serve to conduct the current in any part of its circuit—be they metal, fluid, nerve, muscle, or bone—the same are all, for the time, component parts of *one complete magnet*, which, in all its parts, is subject to the law of polarization, precisely as if it were one magnetized bar of steel. Usually, however, it is sufficient for *practical* purposes to contemplate the circuit as consisting only of that which the current passes through in going from the point where it leaves the positive post and enters into the negative cord, around to the point where it leaves the positive cord and enters into the negative post.

POLARIZATION OF THE CIRCUIT.

I have said, in effect, a little above, that, while the current is running, *the entire circuit is one complete magnet,* which extends from the inner or positive sides of the zinc plates, where the current commences, all the way around to the outer or negative sides of the zinc plates, to which it returns. Viewed in this light its negative pole or end is the battery fluid, next to the positive surfaces of the zinc plates, and its positive pole or end is the brass clamp which, holding the metals together, is in contact with the outer and negative surfaces of the zincs.

But, for practical purposes, it is sufficiently exact to consider the *magnetic circuit* as extending only from the positive *post* around through the conducting cords, the electrodes and the person of the patient to the *negative* post. The negative end or pole of this magnet is the wire end of the cord placed in the positive post, and the positive end or pole is the wire end of the cord placed in the negative post.

But any magnet may be viewed either as one whole, or be conceived as composed of a succession of shorter magnets placed end to end. If we view it as one entire magnet, we call the end in which the magnetic essence is in greatest quantity the *positive* end, and the end where it is in least quantity the *negative* end.

But if we imagine the one whole magnet as being divided up into several sections, then we conceive of each section as a distinct magnet, having its own positive and negative poles. And, all the way through, these sectional magnets will be arranged with the positive pole of the one joined to the negative pole of the next in advance of it.

It is just so in respect to the magnetic circuit of a moving current. The whole circuit, as before remarked, is in reality one long magnet. But in applying the terms *positive* and *negative* in our practice we often view the whole circuit—the one long magnet—as composed of a series of shorter ones, arranged with positive and negative ends in contact; and all the way the current in each section is supposed to be running from the positive pole of the magnet behind to the negative pole of the magnet before.

We consider the circuit, from the positive post around to the negative post, as composed of three magnets, as follows: Magnet No. 1, which extends from the positive post, along the cord and electrode, to the body of the patient, where the positive electrode is placed. The *negative pole* of this magnet is the *wire end of the cord* placed in the positive post, and its *positive* pole in the *positive electrode* placed upon the person of the patient. No. 2, which is composed of the parts of the patient traversed by the current between the two electrodes. Its negative end or pole is the part in contact with the positive pole of magnet No. 1, and its positive pole is the part in contact with the negative pole of magnet No. 3. No. 3 extends from the positive pole of No. 2, through the electrode and along the cord, to the negative post. Its negative pole is the *negative electrode* in contact with the positive end or pole of magnet No. 2, and its positive pole is the *wire end of the cord* in the negative post.

Since in every magnet the magnetic fluid is supposed to be regularly graduated from minimum quantity in the negative end to maximum quantity in the positive end, this is true in respect to the one magnet, consisting of the whole magnetic circuit, as well as in respect to each one of the sectional series. Consequently there must be the same quantity of magnetism in each negative pole of the sections as there is in the positive pole of the section immediately behind it. And the magnetism of the whole circuit between the positive and the negative posts is in its *least* volume next to the *positive post*, and in *fullest* volume next to the *negative post.* If we consider the circuit as divided into two equal halves, the *negative half* is plainly that which joins the *positive post*, and the *positive half* that which joins the *negative post.*

From this it will be seen that what in practice are designated as the positive and negative *posts*, and also positive and negative *poles* or *electrodes* are *not* such *in relation to each other*, but the *reverse* of it; that is to say, the positive *post* is not *positive* in relation to the *negative post*, but is *negative* to it; and the positive *electrode or pole* is not positive in relation to the *negative* electrode, but *negative* to it. The positive *post*, like the positive *electrode*, is called *positive*, because it is the positive end of the sectional magnet next *behind* it. And the *negative* post, as also the negative electrode, is *called negative* because it is the negative end of the sectional magnet next *in advance* of it.

THE CENTRAL POINT OF THE CIRCUIT.

The central point of the circuit—that point which divides between its positive and negative halves—is reckoned, in practice, to be the midway point in the line over which the current passes, in its whole course from the positive post around to the negative post. When the cords are of equal length, this point will always be in the person of the patient, about midway between the parts where the two electrodes are applied. This central point, or "point of centrality," is practically neuter—neither positive nor negative; and upon the two opposite halves of the circuit, the positive and negative *qualities* of the current are in greatest force nearest to the posts, and in least force nearest to the central point. At this point they cease altogether, and the central point is *neuter*.

It may, perhaps, be observed that, in *apparent* contradiction of this statement, the *sensational* effect of the current on the negative half of the circuit is *least* nearest to the positive post, and becomes regularly *greater* as the current advances towards the central point; and that *at* this point it is greater than at any other point between this and the positive post. To relieve this seeming contradiction, it is only necessary to consider that, in fact, the *positive* state on the negative half of the current *does* increase regularly from the positive post to the central point. But that which is the *increase* of the positive state is the *decrease* of the negative state. So it is still true that on the negative half of the circuit, the *negative* qualities *diminish* as we advance towards the central point just as on the positive half, the *positive* qualities diminish regularly towards the central point, as stated above.

THE CURRENT.

The current is that moving electric essence which traverses the circuit. The *course* of the current is always from the positive to the negative. It leaves the machine at the positive post, where it enters the cord which holds the positive electrode or pole. Thence it advances around the circuit, going out from the opposite cord where that connects with the negative post. The forward end of the current is its positive end; the rear, of course, is its negative end. At its forward end it is in its greatest volume. At its rear end the volume is least. At the *central point* of its circuit there is the *mean* quantity—the *average* volume. And because the positive and negative forces on either side exactly balance each other upon the central point, therefore this point is practically neuter—neither positive nor negative.

MODIFICATIONS OF ELECTRICITY.

In the present stage of electric science, the conviction has become very general among experimenters that galvanism, magnetism, faradaism, frictional electricity and the electricity of the storm-cloud are, in their essential nature, one and the same; being diversified in appearance and effects by the different modes and circumstances of their development. This conviction has been reached in various ways; but chiefly, perhaps, by observing the many analogies between the phenomena of these several forces, and also by the fact that each of them can be made to produce or be produced by one or more of the others. But I must forego any detailed discussion of this matter, since my limits will not admit of it, and shall assume that these apparently several agents are but modifications of the same generic force.

There are two other phases or modifications of the electric principle, as I judge them to be, which are not so generally classed here. I refer to the forces of animal and vegetable vitality, as viewed in the next section.

VITAL FORCES—ANIMAL AND VEGETABLE.

Upon these points I must be permitted to offer a few words.

Of the *animal kingdom*, I regard the "nervous fluid" or "nervous influence," popularly so called, as being the very principle of *animal vitalization*—the life force; and that, a modification of the *electric* force. It is, I think, pretty generally conceded at this day that the "nervous influence" is probably electric. There are some alleged facts, and other certain facts, which go far to sustain this view. It is said that if we transfix, with a steel needle, a large nerve of a living animal, as the great ischiatic, and let it remain in that condition a suitable time, the needle becomes permanently magnetized. So, too, if the point of a lancet be held for some length of time between the severed ends of a newly-divided large nerve, that point, as I have heard it affirmed, on what appeared to be good authority, becomes magnetized; although I have not attempted to verify either of these cases by experiment. However, admitting them to be true, the metal is charged with simply the "nervous fluid." But the fact on which I myself chiefly rely for evidence of this identification, being almost daily conversant with it in my practice, is this: *The "nervous influence" obeys the laws of electrical polarization, attraction and repulsion.* When I treat a paralyzed part, in which, to all appearance, the action of the nerve force is suspended, I have but to assume that this force is electric, and apply the poles of my instrument accordingly, and I *bring it in* from the more healthy parts, along with the inorganic current from my machine. Forcing conduction through the nerves, by means of my artificial apparatus, I rouse the susceptibility of the nerves until they will normally conduct the "nervous influence" or electro-vital fluid, as I term it, and the paralysis is removed. Again, if I treat an inflamed part, in which the capillaries are engorged with arterial blood, I have but to assume that the affected part is over-charged with the electro-vital fluid, through the nerves and the arterial blood, and so to apply my electrodes, according to well known electrical law, as tö produce mutual repulsion, and the inflammatory action is sure to be repressed. I manifestly change the polarization of the parts. This thing is so perfectly regular and constant that I am entirely assured, before touching the patient, what sort of effect will be produced by this or that arrangement in the application of the poles of the instrument. If I desire to increase or depress the nervous force in any given case, I find myself able, on this principle, to produce the one effect or the other, at will. Hence, I say, the nervous influence obeys the electric laws, just as does the inorganic electricity. I find this subtle agent not in the nerves only, but also in muscle and blood—more especially in arterial blood. Indeed it seems to pervade, more or less, the entire solids and fluids of the animal system. And wherever it exists, its action is just that of an *electro-vital* force. Examples of this fact will appear further along in the present work. While, therefore, I can not *affirm* the identity of animal electricity and animal vitality, the theory of their identification, to my view, best accords with the manifestations under correct therapeutic treatment, and I am unaware of any established fact to disprove it.

Vegetable vitality, also, I regard as another modification of the electric force. The fact has been proved by repeated experiments, that galvanic currents, passed among the roots of vegetables, causes a quickened development of the plants to a degree that would be deemed incredible by almost any one who had neither seen it nor learned its *rationale*. I have seen it stated, on authority which commanded my credence, that by this process lettuce leaves may be grown, within a few hours only, "from the size of a mouse's ear to dimensions large enough for convenient use on the dinner-table."

The following experiment has been related to me by several different parties, as having been made by *Judge Caton*, of Ottawa, Illinois; and subsequently the same has been confirmed to me by his brother, Deacon Wm. P. Caton, of Plainfield, Illinois. It is said that the Judge had some interesting *evergreens* which appeared to be affected by an unhealthy influence, causing a suspension of growth and withering of branches here and there, until such branches died. So the process went on, terminating after a little time in the death of the trees. In this way he had lost some valuable specimens. At length a very fine and favorite evergreen was similarly attacked. He felt, of course, annoyed by the destructive process, and especially reluctant to lose this particular tree. Probably calling to his recollection something analogous to what I have referred to above, he resolved to try the efficacy of galvanism to reinforce the vitality of the shrub. Having a telegraphic wire extending from the main line in Ottawa to his own residence, he availed himself of this facility, and caused a wire to be passed among the roots of this tree in such a way as to bring the galvanic current to act upon them. It was not long before he saw, to his delight, a new set of foliage starting from the twigs, and after a little time the tree was again flourishing in all its beauty. The electric current had evidently imparted to it a fresh vitality.

To insure the success of such an experiment, a proper regard to polarization must be had, such as is taught in the system presented in this book. There may not have been any attention to this matter in the case just related; but if not, the Judge must have *stumbled* upon the correct application of poles. To have brought the roots under the influence of the wrong pole would have made sure the death of his tree.

Now, although, if taken by themselves, such experiments could not be regarded as *conclu-*

4

sive in favor of the electric nature of vegetable vitality, notwithstanding that this theory best explains the phenomena; yet, when considered in connection with the fact that the nervous fluid of the animal kingdom is evidently a modification of electricity, and probably constitutes the vital force of the animal, the theory of its identification, under another modification, with the vital principle in the vegetable kingdom also, as deduced from experiments like those just adverted to, receives strong confirmation, and is now, I believe, being adopted by many of the best philosophers of the age.

EXTENT OF ELECTRIC AGENCY.

When we have settled upon the position that the electricity of the heavens and of the artificial machine are identical, and that their identity is essentially one with galvanism, magnetism, the electro-vital fluid of animal and the life-force of the vegetable kingdoms, it requires no extravagant imagination, nor remarkable degree of enthusiastic credulity, to suppose that all the forms of physical attraction and repulsion are due, under God, to the diversified modifications of the same all-pervading agent—ELECTRICITY. Indeed, for myself,

I feel no hesitation in expressing it as my belief that electricity, in one phase or another, and controlled only by WILL, is the grand motive-power of the universe. I believe that, in the form of electro-vital fluid, the great Creator employs it as His immediate agent to carry on all the functions of animal life; and that, in respect to voluntary functions, He subordinates it as a servant to the will of the creature, to effect such cerebral action and such muscular contractions as are demanded by the creature's volitions. I am disposed to think that, by the omnipotent power of His will, He controls and uses electricity, in its various modifications, as the immediate moving-force by which He accomplishes all the changes in the physical universe. It is fast becoming a generally-received opinion among modern *savans*, that every body in nature is really magnetic, more or less; and that all visible or sensible changes are but the result of changing poles. Chemical affinities and revulsions are believed to be only the more delicate forms of electrical attraction and repulsion; the ultimate particles of matter, no less than matter in masses, being subject to the control of electrical laws. The imponderable agents, light and caloric, under the ingenious tests of scientific scrutiny, are beginning to give some very decided indications of being simply electric phenomena. Indeed, the doctrine or theory that supposes caloric to be simply *atomic motion* is even now being very generally accepted by the scientific world. And that motion in the atoms of a body which causes in us the sensation of heat is probably electric motion. And permit me to observe that, though the operations of nature seem, at first thought, to be wonderfully complex and mysterious, yet if the views here presented be correct, the marvel is changed; and we are brought to a profound admiration of the *simplicity* of the means by which the Almighty conducts His material operations. A *single* agent made to perform processes so infinitely numerous, diversified and apparently complex! How amazing! Simplicity in complexity!—majestic, like the mind of God.

THEORY OF MAN.

Let the question now be raised—*What is man?* The answer will have much to do with the remedial system which I aim to teach. For this reason it is thus early introduced.

My answer to the above question is as follows: *Man is a threefold being, composed of a body material, a body electrical, and a spirit rational and indestructible.*

Let the elements of this definition be a little amplified:

1. *The material body.* This is composed of various metals, earths, carbon, phosphorus, and gases. I need not go into a representation of their multiplied and curious combinations to form the many parts of the body complete. But these are the ultimate elements; and a most superb and wonderful structure they here compose. Yet, notwithstanding all the manifest skillfulness of its contrivance, and the power of its accomplishment, and the niceness and beauty of its execution, it were a useless display if unaccompanied with the invisible agents which compose the two other grand constituents of man, to wit: the body electrical and the spirit, or mind. Without these, it would quickly fall into decay, as we see it when deprived of them, and would be resolved into its original elements again. But to our gross material bodies the Creator has added,

2. *The body electrical.* By this, I mean that which has commonly been termed "nervous influence," "nervous fluid," "nervo-vital

fluid," and "nervo-electric fluid." I object, however, to each and all of these designations. They are too restricted and specific. They all seem to imply that it is an agent or influence which appertains especially to the *nervous* system; whereas the entire organism is under its pervading force. I do not doubt but its chief action is in and through the nervous system; but it also pervades and, as I think, vitalizes the whole body. The nervous system seems to be created as one principal means for its replenishment,* and to serve as the medium of its ministrations to the body at large. I choose to term it *electro-vital fluid*, or *electro-vitality*. My reasons for so designating it are the following: (1) It is demonstrably electrical in its nature. (2) It appears to be identified, or at least connected immediately, with the vitalization of the body. (3) I wish, by its name, to distinguish it from *mental* vitality, or the vitality of *spirit*. Whether, as a peculiar manifestation of the electric principle, it vitalizes by its own nature and action solely, or whether

* The *process* of this will probably be explained if another edition should be called for. It is given in one of the author's Class Lectures.

it be *charged* with another mysterious element—a *life-force*—and vitalizes by ministering the latter to the material organism, I will not positively affirm. Whichever it be, the name I assign to it seems sufficiently appropriate. But I strongly incline to the theory that this electro-vital principle does itself, by virtue of its own nature, vitalize the system. In other words, I am disposed to think that God makes it the *immediate* agent of vitalization; having constituted it the *vis vitæ* of both the animal and the vegetable kingdoms. Nor does this idea, as I conceive, necessarily conflict at all with the doctrine of *cell-life*, as maintained by the best physiologists of the present day. I also sometimes style this electro-vital element the *body electrical*, because it is certainly an entity, coëxtensive with and, in greater or less force, wholly pervading the visible, material body.

At this point I will take the liberty to introduce, although somewhat digressively, a few thoughts on the DISTINCTIONS OF VITALITY OR LIFE.

There are, as I suppose, the following several kinds of life: (1) *Spirit life;* (2) *Moral life;* (3) *Electric life.*

(1.) There is *spirit* life. And here are to be made several subdivisions.

[1.] *Uncreated* spirit life. This is the life of God. Of the nature of the Divine Essence we know nothing; yet that God is a real, living entity, we do know. My own conviction is that the divine essence and the divine life are identical; that God, a spirit, is necessary, infinite, conscious VITALITY—the voluntary Originator of all existencies besides himself. But as to what is the essential nature of this vitality—this eternal spirit-life—we can have no conception, only that this life is God.

[2.] *Created* spirit-life. And here we make another subdivision.

(*a*) The life of created *immortal* spirit. This is a rational, intelligent entity, representing the spirit of man and of unembodied, created intelligences above him. This spirit God created as it pleased him—"in his own likeness"—a living, indestructible essence; and, as I suppose, its essence and its life the same.

(*b*) The life of created *mortal* spirit, as the spirit of the beast. Of the intrinsic essence of this spirit, we are also necessarily ignorant. Yet, of its attributes we know that it has *consciousness*, *sensibility*, and *will*. Of its life we know as little as of its essence; both of which, however, as I conjecture, are also one and the same—the spirit substance being itself essentially vital.

(2.) We pass next to *moral* life. This life is identical with *holiness*—the very opposite of that defilement that characterizes moral *death*, which is a state of *sin*. But let me again subdivide.

[1.] As to the moral life of *God*, it consists in his infinite moral purity—his *veracity, justice* and *benevolence* or *love*—qualities which, in their combination make up his holiness.

[2.] The moral life of *man, as also of other rational creatures.* This consists in his *sympathy of spirit with God* in respect to those pure qualities which constitute the Divine holiness.

(3.) Finally, there is *electric* or *physical life*. But here again there are varieties.

[1.] There is *animal* life, as of man and the lower animals. This I have already represented as consisting in the electro-vital force.

[2.] *Vegetable* life. This is another modification of the same essential principle—electro-vitality.

But now, to return to the *physical* or *animal*

life of man—the electro-vital element. While this is in such *immediate* relation to the visible body on the one hand, it holds, also, on the other hand, an *immediate* relation to the mental part, both of man and of the other animated beings of earth. It serves to transmit, through the nervous system to the mind, all sensations and impressions from the outer world. It, moreover, receives from the mind the action of its volitions and imaginary conceptions, and conveys through the nerves the impressions or impulsions thus obtained to the various parts of the body, and there secures the fulfillment of the mind's behests. It appears to be only in this way that communication is had between the mind and its outer body. The natures of spirit and of gross matter are so totally unlike, that it seems impracticable for the mind and body to come into *immediate* mutual relation, or to act reciprocally, without the aid of a *medium*— ethereal, semi-material and semi-spiritual, such as is the electro-vital fluid. And the Creator has accordingly provided this mysterious, invisible medium between the two, and thus, in a degree, extended man's likeness to himself by making him *a trinity in unity.*

3. *The mind or spirit.* This is immeasur-

ably the highest and most important constituent of man. His body material may fall back to dust. His body electrical may be reabsorbed in the great ocean of natural electricity that fills the earth and the heavens. But his mind is immortal. His spirit, made in the divine image, lives and acts, thinks and feels, independently of every other existence save Him from whom its being came. While in connection with its visible body, its good or ill, its bliss or woe, has, indeed, much to do with its bodily state. But, when separated from this body, its high and more independent existence is at once asserted; and then its good or ill are determined by its Author only in accordance with the workings and affections within itself. A spiritual and indestructible being like its Creator, it can never cease to be while he exists.

But our present concern is with the mind in its relation to that electro-vital medium between it and the body, and to the body itself. The mind's influence upon both of these lower parts of the entire man is truly wonderful, although perceptible mostly on the material body. Few persons are aware how much the state of the mind affects the bodily health, although the degree is often very great. Yet this is done by the mind's action, first on the electro-vital functions, and through these, by way of the nerves, upon the bodily tissue. Changes in the mental states will, in this way, frequently produce changed polarization in the physical organs, and thus determine infallibly the matter of health or disease. So, too, the condition of the bodily health will often determine irresistibly the mental state. Whatever bodily changes affect the polarization of the electro-vital medium in any part of the organism, do thereby produce corresponding changes in the mind.

These views of the reciprocal action between mind and body, through the medium of the electro-vital element, may serve to explain those psychological wonders exhibited in the cure of diseases by the imagination, as well as in diseases and even death induced by the imagination. I would much like to unfold and illustrate this bearing of the subject; and, also, in the light of it, to show the *philosophy* of one mind acting intelligibly on another mind, with, and even *without*, the aid of the physical organs, as is sometimes seen in the facts of mesmerism. This I have done in my written lectures, for the instruction of classes; but my limits will not admit of it here.

There is another thought which I will offer in this connection. I maintain that all *functional* action of our bodily organism, *ab initio*, is conducted by *thinking mind*, through the medium of organic electricity or the electro-vital fluid. Every organ as a whole, and every life-cell in detail, is charged with this active principle. I believe that every one of them is controlled and guided incessantly in its propagating, organizing and entire functional force by *intelligent mind*, acting through this wonder-working agent—the electro-vital fluid. In respect to our *voluntary* exercises, this organic electrical force is made subject to our own mental activities, and executes its office upon the bodily organism mainly through the medium of the nerves. But, as regards all the *involuntary* functions, I believe that control is exercised *directly* by the omniscient and all-pervading God, although in accordance with his own established laws.

Once more of the *mind* let me remark, that *consciousness, sensation, and will belong to it alone.* The *body* never thinks nor feels; nor does the organic electricity within it. The popular idea, especially with the less educated masses, is that, if a man burn his finger, it is the finger that smarts. But this can not be true. Pain can exist only where consciousness is. And there is no consciousness in the finger, nor in any material part. Only the *mind* is conscious of *existence,* even; and hence only the mind can be conscious of pleasure or pain. If a limb be paralyzed, by interrupting in any way the flow of the electro-vital fluid through its nerves, and thus depriving the *mind* of its medium of communication with it, you may burn that limb to a crisp and the subject will feel no pain. When you burn your finger or break your arm, you disturb the action of the electro-vitality in the injured part, deranging its poles. This electric agent instantly communicates its disturbance along the nerves to the brain, where it reports to the mind and tells where the disturbance is. The conscious mind takes cognizance of the fact and feels distress.

THE LOWER ANIMALS.

It may, by some, be objected that, if we regard sensation as existing only in the *mind,* as affirmed above, then we must concede mind to the lower animal tribes, since they are subjects of consciousness, sensation and will, as truly as ourselves. I admit this necessity, and unhesitatingly take the position, as has been already done in the classification of minds, that the lower animals are in fact endowed with a something higher and more spiritual than their material bodies or their animal vitality—something which bears distinguishing characteristics of *mind.* I would not, however, be understood to say, or to imply, that they possess *all* the characteristics of our minds, even in a rudimental degree. I do not believe they do. My theory does not accord to them either reason or immortality. Yet, in respect to the latter, my views are less decisive, and my utterances usually more reserved. But I think their minds may, and probably do, perish with their bodies. Nevertheless, the existence of consciousness, sensation and will, in any orders, does evidently presuppose some sort of mental constitution. And such mental structure, in them as well as in us, must be distinct from and superior to the animal vitality—compelling service from the latter, and using it as a medium for communicating with the body, and with the outer world in general.

THE VEGETABLE KINGDOM.

As to the vegetable kingdom, there is here, so far as we can discover, only a duality of principle, viz: the material body and a modified phase of electro-vitality. These component parts appear to sustain to each other, in the vegetable, relations quite analogous to those of the corresponding parts in the animal. But here the *mental* part is wanting; and consequently there is no consciousness, sensation, nor will; and the electro-vital action is guided in its elaborate and beautiful operations for the forming and developing of the plant, and in all its vital functions, by the all-pervading mind of God.

NATURAL POLARIZATION OF MAN'S PHYSICAL ORGANISM.

The electro-vital fluid, in the animal economy, is subject to the same principles of polarization as the magnetic current from the artificial machine, or the magnetism of the bar-magnet. In the material organism of man, the great nerve-centers—the brain, the spinal cord, and the ganglions—appear to act the part of fixed magnets, charged with the electro-vital fluid. Indeed, there is much reason to believe that this fluid is elaborated within these nerve-centers—more especially within the brain—from the inorganic electricity of the outer world, which is supplied through the lungs in respiration, and conducted thence to these laboratories by a remarkably interesting process—a process which I have not room here to describe, but which I have drawn out in detail in a manuscript lecture on the circulation of the blood, for my classes, and which may some day see the light. These nerve-centers, viewed as magnets of electro-vitality, require to be regarded as having each a positive nucleus in the interior, on which are ranged the negative ends of the currents which go out from this positive nucleus in every direction to the surface of the medullary organ—so radiating, as it were, from center to periphery. And the nerve-lines and ramifications which issue from these great nerve-centers are polarized evidently in the same way—the electro-vital fluid being disposed with its negative ends to the positive surfaces of the nerve-centers, and its positive or plus ends to the "vital organs," and especially to the surfaces of the organism as a whole. There are many other polarizations in the human system, subordinate to those mentioned above; but I have no room to speak of them in detail.

ELECTRICAL CLASSIFICATION OF DISEASES.

There are two, and only two, primary classes of disease—those in which the electro-vital force is abnormally *positive*, and those where it is preternaturally *negative*. The former class comprises every variety and phase of hypersthenia, and the latter, every sort and degree of anæsthesia, or rather, of azoödynamia. *Inflammation* may be taken as a general representative of the positive or hypersthenic class—those forms of disease in which there is too much electro-vitality, or in which the vital force may be said to be too active. *Paralysis* may stand as a general representative of the negative or azoödynamic class—those in which the vital action is too low or weak.

PHILOSOPHY OF DISEASE AND CURE.

In every part of the animal economy, polar derangements in the electro-vital principle are liable to occur. These derangements are always the real foundation of disease. They may be occasioned by a thousand agencies, which act as the *procuring* cause of disease; but the *proximate* and *sustaining* cause is polar disturbance—derangement of the electro-vital poles. Parts which, in health, are relatively positive, may become negative, and that which should be negative may become positive. Or again, a part, naturally positive to its counterpart, may become *excessively* so, and that which should be relatively negative may become negative to a *morbid degree.*

To correct these polar disturbances and restore the normal polarization, is to *cure the complaint.* This is, under the treatment of most physicians, often accomplished by the use of medicines, and by mechanical or surgical agency. We accomplish it by the proper application of the *poles* of our electrical apparatus. In cases where there is *virus* to be destroyed, or *abnormal growths* to be removed, we also secure the *chemical* action appropriate to these ends by the proper *selection of our current.* It often happens that *mechanical* or *surgical action* is demanded. In many *such* cases, we do not profess to secure normal polarization and consequent cure by means of electricity alone. Yet, in a large proportion of the cases where mechanical or surgical agency is usually thought to be indispensable, we are able to cure by electric action only, since by it we can exert very considerable mechanical force at will; and can also, in many instances, attain much more happily, by means of electricity, the very ends or the *best* ends which would be aimed at by skillful surgical operations.

PRINCIPLES OF PRACTICE.

POLAR ANTAGONISM.

When the conducting cords are of equal length, as commonly they should be, each of the two poles or electrodes produces a polar effect in the patient directly the opposite of that produced by the other. Also, *at any point* in either half of the circuit, if it be within the person of the patient, the polar effect produced is the very reverse of what is experienced at the corresponding point in the other half of the circuit. And further; each half of the current produces a polar effect, at every point in the parts of the patient through which it runs, the same in *kind,* though differing in *degree,* as is produced immediately under the pole or electrode with which it is connected; yet an effect antagonistic to that which is produced under the other pole, or at the corresponding point in the other half of the current.

IMPORTANCE OF NOTING THE CENTRAL POINT.

From the above observations, it will be plain that, when we wish to bring a diseased organ under the influence of the *positive* pole, we must carefully place our electrodes so that none of the organ, or none of the diseased part of it, shall appear on the positive * side of the *central point of the circuit;* it being understood that the current moves as nearly in direct lines as the best conducting medium will admit. Or again, if it be desired to bring a diseased organ, or any extended part of it, under the influence of the *negative* pole, we must first calculate in placing our electrodes about where the central point will come, and then so apply them that no part of the lesion or disease shall appear on the negative * side of the central point; otherwise so much of it as lies on that side will come under the force of the wrong pole, and thus be affected in a way the opposite of what was intended. The characteristic influence of each pole is felt throughout its own half of the circuit.

---

* Study carefully *Polarization of the Circuit*, page 29.

DISTINCTIVE USE OF EACH POLE.

I have said that every disease is preternaturally either positive or negative. I have further said, that the application of either pole to a given part produces an effect the opposite of what would be produced in the same part by a reversal of the poles. The way is now prepared for me to announce THE CENTRAL PRINCIPLE of our system of practice. The reader will bear in mind that all acutely inflammatory or hypersthenic affections are electrically *positive* in excess—having too much vital action—being *overcharged* with the electro-vital fluid; and that all paralytic diseases, or those of a sluggish, azoödynamic character, are electrically *negative*—having too little electro-vital fluid—too little vital action. It is a universal law of electricity that positives repel each other, and that negatives repel each other; but that positives and negatives attract each other. This is a principle of electric action every-where known, where any thing is known on the subject. *We appropriate it practically to therapeutic purposes.* Therefore, when I wish to repress or repel inflammation, which is electrically positive in excess, I put the positive pole to it; or, at least, I bring it under that half of the circuit with which the positive pole is connected, and as near to the pole or electrode as possible. And because two positives repel each other, and also because the direction of the current is always from the positive to the negative pole, carrying the electro-vital fluid with it, either I must withdraw my positive electrode, or that excess of electro-vitality in the diseased part which makes it morbidly positive, and thus produces inflammation, must give way. I *will not* withdraw my positive pole, and therefore the positive inflammation *must* retreat and be dispersed. In treating this case, I will place my *negative* electrode either on some healthy part, or, if there be perceptible anywhere in the system a morbidly negative part, as is often the case, I will place my negative pole there. For example: if I am treating for *nephritis*—inflammation of the kidneys—when I do not perceive any part to be abnormally negative, I manipulate with my positive electrode over the inflamed kidney, having the negative electrode placed at the coccyx—lowest part of the spine. My positive pole repels the positive inflammation from the kidney; or, rather, repels from it that excess of electro-vital fluid which makes it morbidly positive and induces the inflammation, while the negative pole attracts the same towards the coccyx. On its way, it becomes more or less diverted to adjacent nerves; or, if gathered in the healthy part, under the negative pole, it is immediately dispersed by the normal circulation as soon as the electrode is removed. But if I find *a spinal irritation,* say in one or more of the cervical or dorsal vertebræ, and, at the same time, a stomach affected with *chronic dyspepsia,* accompanied with *constipation of bowels,* I will work over the inflamed or irritated spine with my positive pole, because I know from its irritation that there is an excess of electro-vital fluid in the part, making it improperly positive; and, with my negative electrode, I will, at the same time, treat over the stomach, bowels and liver; because I know, from the *inaction* of these organs, that there is a lack of the vital force—a deficiency of the electro-vital fluid—there, and that, consequently, they are too negative. Adopting this method, I accomplish two objects in the same treatment. *First,* my positive pole, applied to the spinal disease, repels from it the excess of electro-vital fluid which was there doing mischief; and, *second*, my negative pole attracts the same, along with the artificial or inorganic electricity, to the stomach and bowels where it is wanted, since negatives attract positives. Or I wish to rouse to action a *torpid liver*. Now, if I find *inflammation, or enlargement* of the spleen, as is commonly the case in *chills and fever*, I place the positive pole upon the spleen, at the left side, just below the false ribs, and the negative pole on the liver, which is best reached immediately below the ribs on the right side, and around backward and upward as far as to the spine. The positive pole repels the excess of electro-vitality away from the positive spleen, and so reduces the improper excitement there, while at the same time it rushes, by attraction, to the negative liver, under the negative pole, and makes that more positive, and so more active. In this way, I change the polarization of the parts, and, in so doing, remove the sustaining cause of the disease. You here perceive that I treat a positive part with the positive pole, so as to repel the excess of electro-vitality from it, and thus repress its excessive action; and that I treat a negative part with the negative pole, so as to attract the electro-vital fluid, along with the current from the machine, to it from under the positive pole, and thus increase the action by making it more positive.

But suppose I do what nearly all of the doctors do, who use electricity with any regard to polarity; that is, if treating acutely inflamed eyes, for example, apply the negative pole to the eyes, thinking thereby to make them more negative; or, if treating amaurosis, apply the positive electrode to the affected parts, thinking thereby to make them more positive! I say, suppose I do this same thing, do you not see that, by the fixed laws of electricity, I necessarily increase the evils that I would remedy? Do you not see that, by placing my negative pole on the already overcharged and inflamed eyes, I attract to them yet more of the electro-vital fluid, and so increase their positive condition and aggravate the inflammation? and that, by presenting my positive electrode to the eyes already more or less paralyzed, I repel what little electro-vitality there was there, and so make the nerves all the more negative and dead? And yet, I repeat it, this is precisely the plan of almost all the men who use electricity in therapeutic practice with any regard to its polarization. They treat a positive disease—rather, a *hypersthenic* disease, (for they seldom know anything of the *electrical* states of diseased parts), with the negative pole, and an azoödynamic disease, which is negative, with the positive pole!—all directly antagonistic to science and success.

But the great mass of physicians, who attempt to treat electrically, have no knowledge either of the electrical condition of the various forms of disease, nor of the distinctive and peculiar effects produced by either pole of the artificial current; and consequently all their use of this powerful agent is entirely empirical—merely haphazard experiment.

I may have raised an inquiry a few moments since which ought to be answered. I said, in effect, that in treating a positive disease, such, for instance, as acute, inflammatory rheumatism or acute pleurisy, I would use the positive pole on the inflamed parts, and the negative pole on either some healthy part or on a morbidly negative part, if I could find such. So, too, I said I would treat a negative disease, such as amaurosis or torpidity of liver, with the negative pole, placing the positive pole on either some healthy or morbidly positive part. The query may have arisen, "By placing the one pole or the other on a healthy part, do you not derange the normal electro-vital action there, disturbing its healthy polarization?" I answer, yes, for the time being, I do; and if this disturbing force were to be steadily continued for any considerable time, the disturbance would produce manifest and serious disease. But then, a pole or electrode, placed on a healthy part, we generally move, or ought to move, more or less, every few moments, which prevents the establishment of any perverted action in the part; and the moment the electrode is withdrawn, the normal polarization and healthy action are resumed.

USE OF THE LONG CORD.

It is often desirable to bring the entire parts of the patient, through which the current is made to pass, under one and the same kind of influence—such as shall make them all more positive or more negative. Especially is this true in many cases where we wish to run through but a *short* space. For this purpose, there is frequent advantage in using conducting cords of unequal length. As my views on this point have been disputed in certain quarters, I will endeavor here to place them in such a light that they shall not be rejected for want of being *rightly understood.*

I have previously remarked* that, for practical purposes, it is sufficiently exact to consider the *magnetic circuit* as extending only from the *positive post,* around through the conducting cords, the electrodes, and the person of the patient, to the *negative post.* We will so regard it at present. This circuit may be viewed as one continuous magnet, made up of several sections or shorter magnets placed end to end—the positive end of the first to the negative end of the second, and the positive end of the second to the negative end of the third. In this arrangement, the negative end of the first section is the negative pole of the one whole magnet, and the positive end of the third section is the positive pole of the whole magnet. The minimum quantity of the magnetism is supposed to be at the negative pole, and the maximum quantity at the positive pole; and the quantity is supposed to increase, by *regular graduation,* from the negative to the positive

---

* *Polarization of the Circuit,* page 29.

pole. This being so, the quantity is *the same* in the positive end of either section and the negative end of the adjoining section, at their point of contact.

Now, in practice, the body of the patient, or so much of it as is embraced between the two electrodes, may be regarded as the *second* section in this magnet; and the cord connected with the positive post, together with its electrode attached, may be counted the *first* and *most negative* section; and the cord connected with the negative post, along with its electrode, may be the *third* and *most positive* section. And if this whole magnet be more and more positive, by regular degrees through all the sections, from its negative to its positive end or pole, then the nearer any given part of it, say the *second section*—the patient's person, may be to its positive pole in the negative post, so much the more *positive* that section or part will be. And the nearer such part or section may be to the negative pole in the positive post, so much the more *negative* it will be. If the cords be of equal length, the central point in the circuit or magnet will be in the second section—the person of the patient, midway between the electrodes; and that section will be charged with the *mean* quantity of the magnetic fluid. The *central point* will hold *exactly* the mean quantity. But if the cord in the *first* section be *two* yards long, and that in the *third* section be *four* yards, then section second—the patient's parts under treatment—will be nearest to the *negative* pole in the positive post, and consequently will be charged with much *less* than the mean quantity of the fluid, and will therefore be made so much the more *negative*. If, on the other hand, the cord in section *first* be *four* yards in length, and that in section *third* be only *two* yards, then the patient's body—section second—will be brought nearest to the *positive* pole in the negative post, and of course be charged with much *more* than the mean quantity of the magnetic fluid, and hence will be made so much the more *positive*.

It is true that the positive and negative poles of section second—the parts of the patient between the electrodes—will not be *reversed* by any such changes in the length or relative positions of the conducting cords; nor is such reversal required in those cases where the use of the *long cord* is indicated. The only change of polarization called for in such cases, is that *all* the parts through which the current is to pass should, in greater or less degree, be affected alike, as being made more positive or more negative. Of course these parts will be so affected in different degrees—those nearest to the *short* cord the *most;* those nearest to the *lony* cord the *least.*

The class of cases where the use of the *long cord* is more especially advantageous, comprises those in which it is desirable to run the current *out* of the patient at the shortest admissible distance from the positive electrode. For example, in treating *cynanche tonsillaris*, (quinsy), if treating with the positive pole in the mouth, we would not wish to run the current further than to the back of the neck; or, if treating externally, we would not wish to carry the negative electrode further from the positive than from side to side. Here the *long cord*, with the negative electrode, would be a special advantage in subduing the inflammation. We would not care to *increase* the inflammatory action, as we should necessarily do on the positive side of the central point, by using cords of *equal* length.

Again, if treating a case of acute *enteritis*—inflammation of the intestines—we would not wish, while treating the abdomen with the positive pole, to increase the inflammation in the lower parts, by using equal cords and placing the negative pole at the sacrum or the coccyx. Neither would we wish to reduce the strength of the lower limbs by carrying the negative pole to the feet. Nor, yet again, would we care to endanger the thoracic viscera by running the current from the abdomen up to the dorsal or cervical vertebræ. The true way, in such a case, would be to connect the negative electrode with a *long cord,* and then to run the current through the inflamed parts, and *out* somewhere from the lumbar vertebræ to the coccyx, by treating over the abdomen with the positive pole, and placing the negative pole on the lower parts of the spine.

As the cords that accompany the machine from the manufacturer are usually cut about two yards in length, every practitioner should supply himself with an extra cord, of at least three yards, to be used as the *long cord.*

THE INWARD AND THE OUTWARD CURRENT.

I have already said that when the conducting-cords are of equal length, as for the most part they should be, the central point of the circuit will be in the person of the patient, about midway between the two electrodes Now, since the current always runs from the positive to the negative pole, and makes its whole circuit in that direction, it will be readily seen that, from the place on the patient where the positive pole is applied, inward as far as to the central point, the direction of the current may properly be said to be *inward;* and that, from the central point to the place of the negative electrode, where the current comes out, its direction may be said to be *outward.* When, therefore, a part is treated with the positive pole, or when the part under treatment appears anywhere between the positive pole and the central point, it is not unusual to say, It is treated with the *inward current.* And when a part is treated with the negative pole, or when it appears between the central point and the negative pole, it is often spoken of as being treated with the *outward current.*

MECHANICAL EFFECT OF EACH POLE.

The *mechanical* effect of the forward end of the current, or that part of it which is under the negative electrode, is to relax, expand and weaken; while that of the rear end, under the positive electrode, is to contract and strengthen. A moving ship disperses the waters at its bow, but draws them in at its stern. The bullet shot from a gun, in passing through a plank, leaves the perforation closed where it enters in, but wide open where it comes out. Thus, in physics, the advance end of a moving body tends to disperse the element through which it is passing, while the rear end tends to its contraction. Analogous to this are the *mechanical* effects of the different ends of an electrical current in the living tissue. When, therefore, we wish to relax a muscle that is unnaturally contracted, as by rheumatism or otherwise, we must bring it under the forward end—the outward current—the negative pole. If we desire to contract ligaments or muscles that are abnormally relaxed, (not *atrophied*), as in prolapsus uteri, we must subject them to the rear end of the current—the positive pole. Parts that are unnaturally contracted are electrically negative in excess, and need to be made more positive. And parts that are unhealthily relaxed are too positive, and should be made more negative. We make a part more positive by applying to it the negative pole, and more negative by applying to it the positive pole. Parts *spasmodically* contracted are acute and positive; those *permanently* contracted are chronic and negative.

RELAXED AND ATROPHIED CONDITIONS.

I alluded, above, to a distinction between a *relaxed* and an *atrophied* condition of an organ. There is such a distinction, which should be carefully observed while treating parts so affected. An atrophied muscle or organ becomes soft and flabby from lack of nourishment. But this condition is not properly one of *relaxation*. It is rather a diminution—a *thinning out* of atoms, by wasting without replenishment. Such a condition is always negative, and requires treatment under the negative pole. On the contrary, relaxed parts, such as appear in prolapsus uteri, and in the sagging down of the diaphragm, with the thoracic and abdominal viscera, exhibit no lack of nutrition or of vital action. Relaxation is a *loosening* of atoms from each other, more or less, without loss of aggregate weight; and implies a condition electrically positive in excess, and calls for treatment with the positive pole.

GENERAL DIRECTIONS OF THE CURRENT.

Negative affections, as a general rule, are best treated with the *upward-running* current—the positive pole being placed at a lower point than the negative. *Inflammatory* affections, and other *plus* conditions, for the most part, should be treated with the down-running current, keeping the negative pole at a lower point than the positive. But these rules admit of frequent exceptions, which every practitioner's experience will soon reveal.

The *downward* current, running *with* the downward and outward course of the nerves, tends to *depletion* and *weakness*, for the reason that it *runs off* from the system the electro-vital fluid. The *upward* current, on the other hand, running *against* the nerves, inward towards their source, feeds the system with fresh electricity, and gives a *tonic* effect. Yet for this purpose, it must not be too long continued, nor of too severe strength, lest it overtask and irritate the nerve-sheaths.

In treating a *paralyzed* organ, the current should commonly be run from a *healthy* part, whether that require it to be directed downwards or upwards. For example: In treating a paralyzed foot or leg, the positive pole should be upon the lower part of the spine—at the coccyx—or even under the sole of the opposite foot. It is best to alternate between these positions. So in treating a paralyzed hand or arm, let the current be run from the upper part of the spine, and frequently also from the opposite hand. With the *negative* electrode, treat all over the paralyzed parts. Yet it is well, in these cases, often to *reverse* the direction of the current for a brief period at the close of the sittings, say one to two minutes, for the purpose of rousing the nervous susceptibility, and to prevent exhaustion from too continuously running off the electro-vital fluid.

TREATING WITH ELECTROLYTIC CURRENTS.

For decomposing and carrying off unnatural growths, as fistula, ficus, glandular enlargements and other tumors, it is often best to dilute the *electrolytic* quality of the galvanic current A B with one or both of the Faradaic currents, as by taking A C or A D instead of A B. But *malignant* and *poisonous* affections, as scirrhus and other varieties of cancer, and also cases of infectious virus, demand continually, or with but occasional exceptions, the primary galvanic current A B. ☞ In treating these malignant affections, the current should be run through as short a distance of *healthy* tissue as possible, yet so as fairly to reach the diseased part. And whether this part be brought, for a given time, under the one pole or the other, the opposite pole should be attached to the *long cord,* so as to throw the central point of the circuit, not in the person of the patient, but out on the long cord, thus bringing the entire organic parts through which the current is passed on one and the same side of the center, and so, under the ruling influence of the sāme pole.

Those diseases which require the chemical or electrolytic currents should, for the most part, be treated under the negative pole, particularly those which need the galvanic current A B, and also old ulcers and *chronic irritation of mucus surfaces.* Glandular enlargements not of scirrhous character, and excrescent growths not poisonous, may often be reduced, and perhaps sometimes cured, under the positive pole. But my own experience, even with these affections, is that it is better to treat them under the negative pole until they come to assume, as sometimes they will, an *acute* state, when the positive pole may be used with success. If, however, it appears desirable to produce a *cauterizing* effect, this must be done by persistent treatment under the negative pole of a strong A B or A C current, and, if the disease be external, with a small pointed electrode.

POSITIVE AND NEGATIVE MANIFESTATIONS.

Acute diseases are to be regarded as electrically positive, and *chronic* affections as negative. The exceptions are rare, if any at all. *Malignant cholera*, which is eminently acute, might by some be considered as an exception. In negative diseases, there is a low degree of electro-vitality. And it has been remarked by careful observers, particularly in the Orient, that cholera rages with greatest destructiveness when no special electric phenomena have for long time appeared in the atmosphere, and when the artificial electrical apparatus could be made to yield its sparks only with difficulty, or not at all. And again, after a thunderstorm, when the electric machine works again freely, the cholera is also found to abate quickly, and sometimes very greatly. The inference drawn from these facts has been that the prevalence of cholera is largely owing to a lack of electricity in the atmosphere, and consequently to a want of the animal electricity or electro-vitality in the system of the patient; and thence it might be concluded that cholera implies a negative condition of the system. I think there is a fallacy in this reasoning. There appears to me to be an unwarrantable assumption in confidently attributing the long absence from the heavens of marked electrical phenomena, and the failure of the electric machine to give its spark, to an unquestioned deficiency of atmospheric electricity. Electrical manifestations take place only when the *plus* and *minus* conditions are existing, in relation to each other, somewhat near, or not very remote; and the visible phenomena appear when the positive and negative rush together, so as to produce a polar equilibrium, But suppose a *plus* condition to exist over a wide region, then, everything being *overcharged*, the visible phenomena would be as rare and as difficult of attainment as if all around were negative. How, then, can it be inferred, with any certainty, from such data, that there is a *deficiency* of electricity, rather than an *excess* of it?

I have not treated a case of cholera; but my

own impression of it is, that in the first stage, or during the "rice-water" discharges, the condition of the system is, as in other acute affections, excessively positive; but that, as the collapse comes on, it rapidly subsides into an intensely negative state, thus assuming the chief characteristic of a chronic condition.

In the above remarks, I would not be understood to indicate any doubt that the prevalence of cholera is often aggravated or mitigated by peculiar electrical states of the atmosphere. It appears altogether probable that such may be the fact; and I should presume that electrical treatment, properly administered, would be found eminently successful in this fearful malady.

Again, in *chronic rheumatism* there might, at first view, seem to be frequent exceptions to the rule last above stated; but the cases alluded to are not such. It is often the fact, during chronic rheumatism, that soreness and severe pain are felt, especially under the presentation of the negative pole, thus showing that these points requre to be treated with the positive pole. But, in such cases, although the general disease of the system be chronic and negative, these sore and severely painful points have, for the time, risen in their electro-vital condition, and so become acute and positive. But when chronic rheumatism is attended with only a *dull* pain, and that chiefly under exercise of the parts, and with little or no increase of pain under an application of the negative pole of the A D current, medium strength, and with no swelling, then the pain, the stiffness and the lameness are all marks of the negative state, and the parts must be treated with the negative pole of the A D current, *strongly* at first, but diminishing in force, from time to time, as the patient becomes relieved.

Alkaline affections—those causing excessive alkaline secretions—are electrically positive. *Acid* or *acidulous* states are negative.

HEALING.

For healing wounds, burns, ulcers, irritation of mucous membranes, and cutaneous eruptions, the A D current is by far the best. *Recent* wounds, contusions and burns are electrically positive. *Old* ulcers and irritations are generally negative.

DIAGNOSIS.

To make a correct diagnosis, it is needful to bear in mind the following general principles:

1. Where the organism is in health, the momentary application to the patient of the negative pole of the double Faradaic current B D—the best for diagnostic use—in good medium strength,* will be directly felt, yet will cause no pain. Whatever *muscular contractions* may be produced for the time, they are harmless, and need not be noticed. Wherever the electro-vital fluid is in *excess*, producing hypersthenia—too much vital action—the part is morbidly *positive;* and, excepting sometimes in the stomach and bowels, the B D current, of medium force, directed to that part under the negative pole, will produce *sharp pain.* But where a current of full medium strength can not be felt under the negative pole, there is a morbidly negative state—a deficiency of vital action—a condition of at least partial paralysis—anæsthesia.

2. In a state of health, different persons will have different degrees of sensibility to the electric current, depending on their varied nervous susceptibility. Again, the same person will be much less sensitive to the current when directed

* By a current of *good medium strength,* I mean one which, in the hands, is ordinarily felt rather strongly, yet not sufficiently so to produce distress.

to the spine, particularly the lower part of it, and to the stomach, than when directed to most other parts. Also, where bones lie near the surface, the periosteum—the membrane immediately investing the bone—is apt to feel more sensibly under the electrodes than the muscular parts. But these variations soon become so familiar to the practitioner that he finds no difficulty in making the proper allowances for them.

In making an electrical examination, the two following questions present themselves to be answered: First, whether anywhere, and, if so, where is there a morbid electrical state in the body of this patient? Second, what is the electrical condition of that unhealthy part? Is it *positive* or *negative?*

These questions being answered, according to the tests just given, the well-instructed practitioner is prepared to go on and treat the patient judiciously, and with success, if success be attainable by any form of medication.

Let me next say, It is best, as a general rule, to make examinations with the *negative pole.* The reason of this is that, since the current is always more energetic under the negative than under the positive pole, it makes itself more sensibly *felt* there than under the positive pole. Indeed, it will commonly be felt even to *painfulness* there, if the part were overcharged and inflamed before. Thus, under the negative electrode, the current readily detects any active disease. But, if we be making the examination with the *positive pole*, as we come upon any point more or less inflamed, the current, quick as lightning, rushes away from such inflamed part to the part under the stationary negative pole, carrying with it, for the time being, more or less of that excess of electro-vital fluid which was in force at the inflamed point; so that *no pain*, perhaps, is experienced there; and thus the disease escapes detection.

I am aware that it has been said by some of our practitioners, with, if I rightly remember, the able discoverer of the grand practical principles of our system, Prof. C. H. Bolles, at their head, that it is not quite prudent to use the negative pole in hand for diagnosis, lest we possibly contract the disease from the patient; since, in that case, the current runs from the patient to the practitioner. They think it safer to use the positive pole in hand; so letting the current run from the practitioner to the patient. There is force in this consideration, without doubt, where the patient is affected with a poisonous or malignant disease. And where any thing of this nature is apprehended, I would never examine with the negative pole in hand. But these cases are commonly so manifest, or so easily determined by colloquial inquiry, that examination with the electric current is rarely if ever necessary. And when the disease is plainly not of a poisonous or infectious nature, I do not think there is any danger to be apprehended from the cause stated. I therefore prefer, as a general rule, to examine with the negative pole; and for the reason given above.

The temperature of the room and the adjustment of apparel should be the same as for treatment. To prevent improper chilliness, the room ought to be of such temperature that clothing is not required for bodily comfort—say, from 70 to 80 degrees, *Fahrenheit*. Seat the patient on a stool or chair, (a stool is most convenient), and yourself at his side, with your machine, ready for use, on a table or bench before him, and a vessel of warm water within easy reach. If the patient be a man we let his trunk be disrobed, giving free access to the back, chest and abdomen. If the patient be a woman, let her be covered with a treating-robe, of which garments the practitioner should keep a supply. They are made much like a lady's plain nightgown; but large and loose, so as to serve ladies of any size, and give ample room to work the electrodes under them. Her skirts should be dropped *below the seat*, so far that their bands shall lie across her lap.

Let us now suppose the machine to be working. We will take the B D current. Let it be of good medium strength. We regulate the strength by the quantity of fluid in the battery, so far as *volume* is concerned, and by means of the plunger as respects *intensity*. The electrodes should be dampened with warm water. Let the *sponge-roll*, [a very thin expansion of sponge, quilted upon a muslin lining, and enveloping one of the tin electrodes], be made the positive pole, and be placed under the coccyx—lowest part of the spine. Then attach the *positive* cord; that is, the cord connected with the *negative* post, to another sponge-roll, to be held in the operator's right hand; or, what is better, attach it to a thin, flexible, metallic wristband, (brass is good, but metallic lace—such as is used in trimming *regalia*, is best), underlaid with wet muslin, and fastened around the right wrist. This brings the operator's hand into the circuit as the negative electrode or pole. Next, pass a moist, warm sponge all over the patient's back. Now, before the back becomes dry, press the points of two fingers firmly, yet not uncomfortably, upon the back of the neck at the base of the skull; thence move gradually downward, by frequent touches of the same firm but gentle character, keeping one finger on each side of the spinous processes, until the whole length of the spine has been, in this manner, passed over. If sharp pain or soreness be felt at any point, *note* that point; there is inflamed irritation there. Then return up to the right or left shoulder, and pass, in like manner, by frequent touches with one or two fingers, over all parts of the back on that side of the spine, down to the hips. Then, in the same way, examine the shoulder and back on the other side of the spine, noting, as before, every point, if there be any, where soreness and pain appear. After this, pass over the entire neck, then over the front parts of the thorax and abdomen, down to the pelvic bones, everywhere watching for soreness and pain. Next, go to the head. Wet the hair through to the scalp, (because dry hair is a bad conductor,) and change to a *very soft* B C current. Then go over all the head in the same manner as over the neck and trunk. Better *reverse* the poles on the head, by transposing the cords in the posts, so as to make the manipulating hand the *positive* pole. The head is, or ought to be, extremely sensitive. You need not do this, however, if the negative pole can be received on the head without discomfort, as it sometimes can be. Commence on the cerebrum, and then pass to the cerebellum.

If, in the examination of the spine, the practitioner finds it uncomfortable to bear in his fingers a current of sufficient strength to be distinctly felt in that part of the patient, he may use the side-sponge cup on the spine. But let him *never use a current on another person* which he does not first apply to his own nerves, so as to know its intensity. Indeed, if one prefer to use the side-sponge cup through the whole process, he can do so; although there is advantage in using the fingers, since, by their concentrated impressions, he is more sure to detect disease than by the broader face of the sponge cup.

☞ Now, wherever there is found *soreness* or *lancinating pain* under the touch, it is sure that the part is preternaturally *positive*—more or less so, according to the degree of painful irritability. On the other hand, if there be found a part evincing much *less* than the usual sensibility found in the *healthy* corresponding part of other patients, it may safely be pronounced torpid or paralytic, more or less. It lacks sufficient electro-vitality—is improperly *negative*, and needs to be treated with the negative pole.

It will often happen that diseased action is found in parts where the patient was entirely unaware of its existence until the prăctitioner's fingers or other electrode revealed it. Again, it will sometimes be found that there is no disease whatever in parts where the patient supposed disease to be active. But when we find patients to be especially nervous, it is not always best to tell them immediately just what our examinations have revealed to us—how severely or how little we think them diseased. It is sometimes better to humor, more or less, the patient's own views for a time; lest, by exciting him or her, we make a difficult case out of one that might have been mastered with comparative ease. In this matter discretion should guide us.

But let me say farther, what I deeply feel, that neither do I think it right to *persistently* conceal from patients, especially those who are dangerously affected, a knowledge of their true condition. In my opinion, physicians often unwittingly incur an awful responsibility in this way, wronging their patients in the most vital and momentous of all interests—the interests involved in a due preparation for death. I believe the true way, in every such case, is for the physician himself, in a kind and soothing manner, to reveal to the patient, little by little, if need be, what he really thinks, or to ask the patient's pastor, or some other calm and judicious person to do it for him. I believe the visits of a discreet and affectionate pastor, or, in the absence of a pastor, of some other mild and Christian friend, to the bedside of the sick is, nine times in ten, not only no embarrassment to the patient's recovery, but positively favorable to it, and ought to be habitually encouraged, rather than restrained, by medical practitioners.

PRESCRIPTIONS.

PRELIMINARY REMARKS.

The author wishes to caution the reader not to rely merely on the forms of treatment here prescribed, but to study thoroughly the principles taught in the preceding pages, until he shall have mastered them, and can judge for himself of the correctness of these prescriptions. It should be remembered, however, that the diseases here considered are viewed in their *simple* or *uncomplicated* states. Where complications exist, the treatment must be modified according to the judgment of the practitioner.

In these instructions, it is always to be understood that the treatment prescribed is with *cords of equal length*, except when the *long cord* is especially mentioned.

In most of the local diseases here named, particularly those which are electrically *negative*, it is desirable to supplement the local treatment prescribed with occasional *general tonic* treatment, where, in the judgment of the practitioner, it can be given without detriment to the local affection.

In all treatments, the electrodes should be moistened with warm water.

GENERAL TONIC TREATMENT.

Take the B D current, (A D is very good), of fair medium strength. Place the sponge-roll, N. P. [Negative Pole], at the coccyx—lowest point of spine—and manipulate with side-sponge cup, P. P. [Positive Pole], from the feet all over the lower limbs to and about the hips; occupying three or four minutes, or less. Then remove the N. P., substituting for the sponge-roll the end-sponge cup, and place this upon the spine at the lower part of the neck. Now manipulate with side-sponge cup, P. P., over the trunk generally, from the lower to the upper parts; giving special attention to the spinal column by treating it somewhat more than other parts. Treat the trunk some five to eight minutes. Next, keeping the N. P. still upon the back of the neck, treat with P. P. over the hands and arms, up to and about the shoulders. Treat here two or three minutes.

It has been customary, for the most part, in giving general tonic treatment, to make the P. P. stationary—placing it successively at the feet, the coccyx and the hands—and to manipulate above it with the N. P. But the better way is as directed above. The object is to reinforce the main nerve-lines and centers with electricity from without. The nerves branch off from their centers—the brain, the spinal cord, the ganglions, and the great plexuses—and run, in general, downward and outward from the trunk lines, in a manner somewhat analagous to the branches and twigs of an inverted little tree. If we place before us such a shrub, with the root upward and the branches pointing downwards, and then draw lines from the lowest point of the lowest twig to the outer ends of all the branches surrounding the main trunk, we shall see that our lines, instead of running in the general directions of the limbs, will, for the most part, run *across* the twigs. But, if we draw our lines from the outer extremities of the branches and twigs up to the root, or near to the source of the trunk, we will find the lines, in the main, running nearly parallel with the branches. Now, let us substitute for this inverted tree the nervous system of a man, and remember that the electric current moves from the positive to the negative pole as nearly in straight lines as it can where there are good conductors, such as the nerves and muscles, and it will at once appear that, in treating the lower limbs, if we place our N. P. at the coccyx, and then manipulate with P. P. over the feet and legs, our electric lines are running from all the surface extremities of the nerve ramifications, wherever the P. P. is moving, directly into and along these fine ramifications, and, through the larger nerve-branches, up to the stationary N. P. Or, if we treat the *trunk* of the body by placing the N. P. on the spine, near its upper end, and then manipulate with P. P. from the lower part upward over the back, sides, abdomen and chest, our current strikes into the surface extremities of the nerves at every point where the electrode touches, and makes its way upwards, along the nerve-lines, to the great spinal cord under the N. P.—thus replenishing with fresh electricity all the ganglions, plexuses and nerve-trunks along the way. But if P. P. be made stationary at the lower end of the section under treatment, and we manipulate over the parts with the N. P., the current strikes from

P. P., across the nerve branches and comes out at their surface extremities wherever the negative electrode moves—so reaching but indirectly and imperfectly the trunk-lines and their centers.

COMMON COLDS.

Take the B D Faradaic current—moderate strength. If the affection be mainly in the head, give,

1*st.* *A face bath.* Let an earthen wash-basin, nearly filled with tepid water, be placed on a table or chair before the patient, he holding the sponge-roll [See page 89] N. P. in his hands. Now let him bury his face in the water as long as he can hold his breath. At the instant after his face is in the water, drop into the water the tin electrode P. P. Repeat this process as often as he recovers his breath, some eight, ten or a dozen times.

2*d.* Place the sponge-roll N. P. in the hands as before, and, making an electrode P. P. of your own hand, in the manner directed for *diagnosis*, clasp the nose of the patient between your thumb and finger, moving them up and down along the sides of the nose, and on the nose between the eyes, about five minutes.

Repeat the above forms twice or thrice a day.

If there be hoarseness, or cough, or stricture of lungs, or soreness of chest, place N. P., with *long cord*, upon back of neck, and treat with P. P. over the front part of neck and breast, and wherever upon the thorax stricture or soreness appears.

If there be a feverish condition of the system, attended, perhaps, with pain in the head, place P. P. on the spine, a little below the cranium, and treat with N. P., *long cord*, all the way down the spine, and over the entire back, sides, thorax and abdomen. In this case let the current be rather mild, and be continued for a considerable length of time, with the view of bringing out perspiration. It is *best* that the patient should receive treatment in bed, perfectly protected from any cool air that might restrain or check perspiration. In these cases, I not unfrequently treat with a light B D current a full hour, unless perspiration start freely in shorter time, working over the trunk and limbs generally. But, while treating over the lower limbs, the P. P. should be upon the hypogastric flexus, at the "small of the back." Treat once or twice a day until relief appears.

After the stricture and soreness of the lungs are removed, and the general febrile action is suppressed, it is desirable to give a *general tonic treatment.*

CEPHALAGIA. (*Headache.*)

1. "*Nervous headache.*" Take the B D current—moderate force. Place P. P. on back of neck, just below the brain, and manipulate with side-sponge cup, N. P., all the way down the spine and over the back.

It may often be necessary to apply the P. P. directly to the suffering part of the head. In that case, take the soft Faradaic current B C. If the fluid in the battery cell be fresh, use very little—just enough to reach well the platina plate and make the machine run. Wet the hair thoroughly through to the scalp, where the electrode is to be applied. Seat the patient on N. P., or let him hold it in both his hands, (the former is the better way), and treat lightly over the affected parts of the head with P. P. Treat five to ten minutes, as may be required, and if the pain returns, repeat the treatment. Only a very light current can be safely applied directly to the brain, and that an *induced* Faradaic current.

2. *Sick Headache.* The *procuring* cause of this distressing disease is involved in considerable mystery. It seems, however, to be largely dependent on the secretion and discharge into the duodenum of an improper quantity of bile, and an irregularity in the peristaltic action of the upper part of the bowels, particularly of the duodenum, in which that action more or less is *reversed*, and thereby throws the biliary fluid up, through the pilorus, into the stomach. After a time, the stomach becomes nauseated by its accumulation; and the head, through nervous sympathy, is rendered electrically positive in excess, and thus is made to ache. Yet there are certain characteristics of the disease which this view does not satisfactorily explain, and which must remain unexplained until advancing science shall reveal to us more perfect light.

When this disease has become habitual and periodic, it is very obstinate, and requires persistent treatment—often for several months.

Take the B D current, with moderate force. Place the N. P. on the spine, immediately above the kidneys, and treat with P. P. over the stomach and the duodenum, (lying transversely just below the stomach), three to five minutes. Treat in this manner about twice a week.

It may sometimes be necessary to treat the head directly. If so, after the treatment above prescribed, add that prescribed for the head directly, in *nervous* headache, with this difference, viz: instead of seating the patient on the N. P., or placing the same in his hands, pass it over the stomach and duodenum, unless the former may be already too positive. In that case, let the N. P. be at the seat.

DEAFNESS.

The prognosis is very uncertain. This infirmity is often cured by our system, even when of long standing; and often, again, the treatment fails. The uncertainty arises from the difficulty in determining the exact pathological derangement.

Take the A D current, mild force. Introduce the ear electrode as the N. P. when the disease is of long standing, or as the P. P. when it is of recent origin. Apply the opposite pole to the back of the neck. Treat five to eight minutes, once a day for three or four days, and afterwards three times a week. If no success appears within three weeks, it will probably be vain to expect it afterwards.

NOISES IN THE HEAD.

Treat the same as for deafness.

INFLAMED EYES.

If the disease be recent and acute, (but not infectious), as from sewing or reading by lamp light or other irritation, take the C D current, of moderate force. Treat with the eye-bath, filled with tepid water, having the eye open in the water. Make the bath the P. P., and place the N. P. on the spine at the upper dorsal vertebra. Treat each eye three minutes daily.

If the disease be acute and *infectious*, use the A C current some four to six times, and then change to A D. Apply the current as directed above.

If the disease be chronic, or the lids granulated, treat with A D, *very mild* current, applying the eye-bath, N. P., to the eyes, and place the P. P. upon the spine, at the top of the back. Treat each eye three to five minutes three times a week.

In cases of simple inflammation, (not infectious), and that chiefly or entirely in the lids, it is often quite as well or better to treat over the closed lids with the finger, holding the sponge-roll P. P. in the same hand.

AMAUROSIS. (*Paralysis of the optic nerve.*)

Use B D current, moderate force, three or four times, and then change to C D. Apply the eye-bath, N. P., to the eye, and sponge-cup P. P. upon one of the upper dorsal vertebræ. Treat three to five minutes on each eye, three times a week.

STRABISMUS. (*Discordance of the eyes.*)

If neither of the *rectus* muscles have been cut and cicatrized, and if the deformity be not congenital, it may ordinarily be cured.

Take B D current, with small pointed electrodes. If the eye be turned *inward*, insert P. P. in the outer angle of the eye, so as to bear upon the *rectus externus*, and N. P. in the inner angle, so as to bear on the *rectus internus*. Let the current be of what force the patient can bear. Withdraw the electrodes frequently, to rest the eye, and then reapply them. Apply the current in this manner six to ten or twelve times at a sitting. The eye will soon become inflamed, but the inflammation will quickly go down. Treat daily, or on alternate days, as the eye can bear. After treating some ten or twelve times, if the organ does not come into place let it rest a week, and then resume the treatment as before.

If the eye be turned *outward*, treat in the same manner as directed above, except that in this case, the P. P. must be inserted in the *inner* and the N. P. in the *outer* angle.

CATARRH. (*Acute.*)

If in the head, treat as prescribed for common colds in the head. If in the throat, place N. P. somewhere on the dorsal vertebræ, and treat with P. P.—tongue instrument—in the mouth about five minutes, and then with end-sponge cup externally upon the affected parts as much longer. Use the B D current, in good medium strength, twice a day.

CATARRH. (*Chronic.*)

If in the head, first give *face-bath*, as in common colds, except with *reversed poles* and changing to the A D current, *very mild* force. If in the throat or bronchial tubes, place the P. P. of the A D current, with *long cord*, on the back of the neck or in the mouth, and treat with N. P., *soft* current, upon the affected parts, eight or ten minutes.

Repeat treatment about three times a week.

DIPHTHERIA.

Use the A D current, strong force. Place the N. P., *long cord*, upon the lower cervical vertebræ, and then treat, *first*, with the *tongue* instrument, P. P., in the mouth, as far back on the tongue as can be borne, three to five minutes. *Next*, manipulate with sponge-cup, P. P., or the tin electrode filled with sponge, over all the front parts of the neck and throat, down to the chest, five to eight minutes.

Treat as often as once in two or three hours.

APHONIA. (*Loss of voice.*)

This affection requires treatment variously, as it depends on one or another procuring cause.

If it be the result of recent "cold," inducing acute catarrhal irritation in the larynx, treat *first* as for *common cold*, and *close* the sitting as follows: Place N. P., *long cord*, of A D current, in good medium force, upon back of neck or in the mouth, and treat three to five minutes, twice a day, with P. P., over the front parts of the air pipe in the neck; mostly over the *larynx*—Adam's apple.

If it be from paralysis of the larynx, treat with B D current, rather strong force; placing P. P., *long cord*, on back of neck or in the mouth, and work with N. P. over the *larynx*, and somewhat over the air tube of the neck generally. Treat three to five minutes, daily.

If, as is sometimes the case, the difficulty proceeds from a relaxation of the diaphragm, with general sagging down of the thoracic and abdominal viscera, so as to draw upon the trachea, then treat the whole trunk tonically, using the B D current. Place the N. P. low on back of neck, and treat with P. P. over the abdomen and thorax, and especially all around the edge of the diaphragm—along the lower line of the false ribs. Treat with medium strength of current, ten minutes, three times a week. The aim is to contract all the relaxed parts, so to relieve the larynx from the strain upon it.

CROUP.

Treat croup, whether membranous or spasmodic, much the same as is prescribed for diphtheria, only, in the latter part of the form, treat less.

ASTHMA.

Use the A D current, medium force. Treat with P. P. over the shoulders and between the scapulæ, and with N. P. in front upon the lungs, heart and diaphragm. Treat five to ten minutes, daily, for three or four days; after that, three times a week.

HEPATIZATION OF LUNGS.

Take A D current, pretty strong force. Treat in front, over the lungs, with P. P., moving N. P., *long cord*, on spine from neck to near the kidneys; that is, over all the dorsal vertebræ. If the current be severely painful, moderate it to endurance. Treat six to ten minutes twice a day.

PNEUMONIA.

Take B D current, forceful as the patient can bear, and treat briefly—say five to seven minutes, several times a day, until relief is experienced.

Place N. P., *long cord*, low on back of neck, and move P. P. over all the upper part of the lungs. Then remove N. P. to the lower dorsal vertebræ, just above the kidneys, and treat with P. P. over the lower part of the lungs. If typhoid symptoms attend, follow the above with placing P. P., medium force, on back of neck, close below the cranium, and N. P. at coccyx, two or three minutes.

PULMONARY PHTHISIS. (*Consumption.*)

After tubercles have been formed *extensively* in the lungs, and have *softened down* over considerable area, carrying down the pulmonary tissue with them into a state of pus, there is commonly but little hope of successful treatment. But where they are restricted to comparatively small extent, and no ulceration exists, they may be decomposed and absorbed away, or be thrown off in expectoration, and the affected parts be healed.

If the case be a *recent* one, and acute fever, combined, perhaps, with more or less inflammation, appear in the lungs, use the A C current, in moderate force, yet all the patient can bear without special distress. Place N. P., *long cord*, upon the upper dorsal vertebræ for treating the upper part of the lungs, or upon the lower dorsal vertebræ for treating their lower part. Then pass P. P. over all the affected parts. Treat in this manner five to eight minutes, daily, until the *inflammation* is suppressed, which will be indicated by an abatement of the extreme sensitiveness and lancinating pain under the electrode. Then, if *feverish* action continue high, remove the N. P. to the coccyx, or to the lower part of the sacrum, taking the B D current, *mild* force, with cords of *equal length*, and treat, as before, with P. P. over the affected parts, and also over the thorax generally, and along down the spine to the lower dorsal vertebræ. Continue this treatment ten to fifteen minutes, daily, until the fever is removed, or nearly so. For this part of the treatment, it is best to use the hand as the P. electrode, and to diffuse the current over the whole palm of the hand wherever special soreness appears. It is better, also, that the patient receive the treatment in bed, secure from any chilliness or current of air, so as to facilitate perspiration.

If the case be one of long standing, and more or less of *pus*, or *pus* and *tubercles*, be raised in coughing, take the A D current, with equal cords and *very* mild force. Reduce the quantity of battery fluid if necessary.

Now place P. P. at the coccyx and treat with N. P., (the hand is here much the best), over all the diseased parts. Change occasionally by removing P. P. to back of neck with *long cord.* The object is to bring the diseased parts under a very light force of the A D current, such as is especially healing in old ulcers and chronic irritation. But if this action should at any time *increase* fever or inflammation in the lungs, the poles must be reversed for one or two treatments. In this stage of the disease, treat ten to twelve or fifteen minutes, daily, for three or four days, and after that, three times a week.

NEURALGIA AND RHEUMATISM OF THE HEART.

If *neuralgia*, use B D current; if *rheumatism*, use A D. In either case, treat the heart with P. P., moderate force, placing N. P. at lower dorsal or upper lumbar vertebræ. Treat five to eight minutes, daily, until relief is gained.

Rheumatism of the heart may be distinguished from *neuralgia* by its occasioning irregularity in the cardiac contractions, commonly a sense of soreness and pain under pressure by the hand, and often perceptible enlargement of the organ, which neuralgia does not, and also by its pains being more constant—less fitful—than those of neuralgia.

ENLARGEMENT, OR OSSIFICATION OF THE HEART.

Treat these two affections in the same way. Take the A D current, moderate force. Place N. P. at the coccyx, or alternately there and, with *long cord*, on the spine opposite to the heart. Manipulate with P. P. over the heart. Treat five to eight minutes, three times a week.

PALPITATION OF THE HEART.

This is commonly a symptomatic or sympathetic affection—*rarely* idiopathic—and disappears on cure of the disease from which it proceeds. It usually denotes nervous weakness, and often general debility. *General tonic treatment* is indicated, as far as can be given without interfering with the proper treatment of any local affections on which the palpitation depends.

TORPID LIVER.

Take A D or B D current, full medium force. Treat with N. P. over the liver, at the right side, immediately below the short ribs, and thence backward and a little upward, as far as to the spine, holding P. P. on the left side, close under the ribs, for about four to six minutes. Then remove P. P. to the spine, on back of neck, two or three minutes. Next, go with the P. P. to coccyx two or three minutes; continuing, as at first, to manipulate with N. P. over the liver. Let the whole treatment occupy some eight to twelve minutes. Repeat the sittings about three times a week.

HEPATITIS. (*Inflammation of Liver.*)

Use the B D current, with what force the patient can bear. Place N. P. at the coccyx, and also somewhat on the trunk, opposite to the inflammation. Then manipulate with P. P. over the inflamed and sore part. Treat five to eight minutes, once or twice a day.

ENLARGEMENT OF LIVER.

Take A D current, with medium force. Place N. P., some three to five minutes, on left side, over the spleen; and then as much longer at the coccyx. Manipulate with P. P. over the liver. Treat about three times a week. If the enlargement be recent, it will subside; if of long standing, its restoration will be slow, and somewhat uncertain.

BILIARY CALCULI. (*Gravel in Liver.*)

Take A C current, strong as can be borne; and treat the inflamed and painful part with P. P., while N. P. is upon the right end of the duodenum. Treat eight to ten minutes, daily.

INTERMITTENT FEVER. (*Ague and Fever.*)

Use the A D current. First, give *general tonic treatment.* (See page 95.) Then close the sitting with a *strong* current, running from spleen to liver—P. P. upon spleen, in the left side, just below the ribs, and N. P. upon liver—best reached in the right side, close under the ribs, and around backward and a little upward as far as to the spine. The spleen is morbidly positive, and probably enlarged, while the liver is too negative. Treat spleen and liver in this transverse manner about five minutes.

If the chills occur on alternate days, treat on the intervening days; if every day, treat about two hours before the chill is expected.

NEPHRITIS. (*Inflammation of Kidneys.*)

1. *Acute.* If the urinary secretion be *reddish* and *scant*, with or without sedimentary deposit, let the inflammation be regarded as *acute;* and use upon it the B D current of good medium strength, or a little more, if the patient can bear it. The pain from the current will probably subside somewhat, and perhaps altogether, under treatment. Place N. P. at the coccyx, and manipulate over the inflamed and sore parts with P. P. Treat five to eight minutes, twice a day, if the case be recent, or once a day, if it be of some weeks standing.

2. *Chronic.* If it be an old case, and attended with a brownish or a brickdust-like sediment in the urine, it may be considered *chronic*, and should be treated with a moderate A D current, once in two days. Place P. P. at the coccyx, and treat with N. P. over the affected kidneys. There may be no sense of soreness or swelling, but *dull* pain. Treat six to ten minutes. But if the inflammation should rise to an active or acute state, *reverse the poles.*

RENAL CALCULI. (*Gravel in the Kidneys.*)

Take the A C current, of considerable force. Place N. P. low upon the bladder, and treat with P. P. upon the inflamed and painful point five to eight minutes, once or twice a day. If treating twice a day, continue not more than five minutes at a time.

DIABETES. (*A Kidney Disease.*)

This disease occurs in two forms—*diabetes insipidus* and *diabetes mellitus.* In the first named form, the disease is readily cured. In the latter, it is very formidable, and is rarely, if ever, cured by medicines; especially when of long standing. In this latter variety of the disease, the urea is absent from the urine, and in its place is found more or less of sugar—often large quantities: Dunglison says 2½ oz. in a pint.

The electrical state of the disease, in both of these forms, is negative in excess.

1. *D. insipidus.* Use the B D current, of moderate force. Place P. P. at the coccyx or on the upper dorsal vertebra, or on both in alternation, which is better, and treat over the

kidneys with N. P. five to eight minutes, once a day for three or four days. If this should fail to cure, (as it seldom will), go on with the same treatment three times a week.

2. *D. mellitus.* Take the A D current, of *mild* force. Place P. P. as in *d. insipidus*, and treat the kidneys with N. P. about five to eight minutes, three times a week; supplementing this with *general tonic treatment*, once or twice a week.

Be patient and persevering. In bad cases, months will be required to effect a cure; but persistent effort, as above prescribed, will rarely if ever fail, unless the vital force is nearly expended.

DYSPEPSIA.

This is one of the most difficult of diseases to control by any of the ordinary modes of medical practice; and yet, under judicious electrical treatment, it is one of the surest to yield. The disease assumes various phases in different persons, and at different times in the same person, requiring varied treatment.

The pain, after eating, is severe; exhalations of air, apparently from the inner surfaces of the stomach and bowels, or of gas from their decomposing contents, are large—often enormous. The stomach is much of the time acid, and, in some cases, sensibly cold, ejecting often a cold mucus. The bowels are habitually constipated. The patient is nervous, irritable, and subject to great depression of spirits. In this stage or phase of the disease, there is a negative condition of the digestive apparatus generally. Treat with the A D current, in mild force, and expect the case to require considerable time. But, since there is no approach to uniformity among patients, no approximation to definite time can be stated. Give *general tonic treatment*, (page 95), three times a week, and close each sitting with local treatment, having P. P. at the coccyx, and manipulating some five minutes with N. P. over the entire front parts of the abdomen and thorax, and over the liver.

It is sometimes found, in old cases, that there is no sensible acidity of stomach; but a *pyrosis*—a burning sensation in the stomach, or a little above, in what is usually termed "the pit of the stomach." Treat this about three minutes with the P. P., strong force; moving N. P., *long cord*, over the lower dorsal vertebræ.

ACUTE DIARRHŒA.

Take B D current. Place N. P., *long cord*, upon the lumbar vertebræ and sacrum, moving it often along the spine, from a position opposite to the umbilicus down to the coccyx; and treat with P. P. over the abdomen, and more especially wherever pain or sensations of uneasiness appear. In severe cases, treat several times in a day—once in two to three hours, if need require, three to five minutes at a time. Use current of full medium strength, if the patient can bear it.

CHRONIC DIARRHŒA.

Take A D current, of *very mild* force. Place P. P. at the feet, and treat with N. P. over the lower limbs *briefly;* then over the bowels and stomach, both front and rear, some three to five minutes; then pass up with N. P. over the anterior parts of the chest, two or three minutes; and, next, place N. P. low on the back of neck, with P. P. still at feet, two or three minutes. Treat in this manner once daily.

If at any time the bowels should become unusually flatulent, and evacuations should increase in frequency, change the treatment. Place N. P. at back of neck, as before, and treat about five minutes with P. P. (force increased to *moderate* current) over the abdomen, daily, from one to three days, as may be necessary. After this, resume treatment as first above prescribed.

COLIC—*of whatever kind.*

Use A D current, pretty strong force. In severe cases, introduce the rectum instrument N. P., *long cord*, or in mild cases, place sponge-roll N. P., *long cord*, at coccyx, and treat with P. P. over all the abdomen, three to five minutes. It may be repeated, if necessary, in thirty minutes.

CHOLERA MORBUS.

Keep the patient still as possible on his back. Use A D current, strong force. Place N. P., *long cord*, at coccyx, and treat with P. P. over abdomen, five to ten minutes, and repeat, if necessary, in thirty to sixty minutes. If there be cramps, touch the contracted muscles with the P. P., for a few moments, without disturbing N. P.

CHOLERA.—(*Malignant.*)

As in cholera morbus, keep the patient on his back, still as can be. Use A D current, *full medium strength.*

In the early stage, or during the "*rice-water*" discharges, and down to the time of collapse, treat the abdomen and thorax with P. P., having N. P., *long cord,* on back of neck—not too near the head. After treating so a few moments—say four to six minutes—remove P. P. to the back, and pass it along close upon each side of the spinous processes from the lower lumbar up to about the middle of the dorsal vertebræ. Continue this about three or four minutes.

If *cramping* accompany the vomiting and purging, carry the P. P. a part of the time to the muscles in spasm, leaving N. P. still at the back of neck, with *long cord.*

Repeat the above processes as often as once an hour until symptoms improve. Then reduce their frequency as the case will admit of.

In the state of collapse, place P. P., *long cord,* at the coccyx, and manipulate with N. P. over the entire trunk and arms; bestowing a larger share of treatment along up the spine than elsewhere. Then remove P. P., *long cord*, to feet, and work with N. P. all over the lower limbs and hips. Treat in this stage of the disease some six or eight minutes at a time, and repeat it as the case seems to demand—once in thirty minutes to once in two, four or six hours, until improvement or death shall ensue. (See page 81.)

DYSENTERY.

Treat exactly as in *acute diarrhœa*, except that P. P. should be moved more over the *colon* and *rectum* than in diarrhœa.

CONSTIPATION OF BOWELS.

This disease may proceed from either a *negative* condition—a state of *atony* from lack of nutrition, or a *partial paralysis* of the bowels—or from a *positive* condition—a state of *relaxation* and consequent weakness of the muscular tissues of the bowels. In either of these cases, the peristaltic action of the intestines becomes enfeebled, and constipation ensues.

In either case, use the A D current, of medium force. In the first-mentioned case, place P. P. at back of neck, or in the mouth with tongue instrument, and treat with N. P. over liver, stomach and bowels; or place N. P. at the anus. Treat so five to eight minutes.

In the second-specified case, place N. P. at back of neck or on the dorsal vertebræ, and treat with P. P. over the bowels five to eight minutes.

In both cases, repeat the treatment daily until relief is afforded. Or, if the case be *chronic*, treat daily for three or four days, and, after that, three times a week. It is well also to give *general tonic treatment* as often as once a week. The patient should be urged to retire and *invite* an evacuation regularly, about the same hour daily, whether success attend it or not.

HŒMORRHOIDS. (*Piles.*)

If the case be recent, take the B D current; if old, take A D. Place the patient in a recumbent position, and let the rectum instrument, P. P., be introduced, *wet.* Manipulate with N. P. along the spine upon the dorsal vertebræ. Where there is *prolapsus ani*, the sponge-roll, placed at the anus, may be used instead of the rectum instrument, particularly for the first few treatments.

RHEUMATISM. (*Acute Inflammatory.*)

First ascertain if the kidneys be morbidly positive—urine scant and too highly colored. If so, as is commonly the case, begin with the B D current, good medium force. Place N. P. at the pelvis, and treat over the kidneys with P. P. some three or four minutes. Let this be the commencement of every treatment until *this* difficulty is corrected.

Next, change to A D current. If the disease be located in the hips or lower limbs, put the feet in warm water with the tin electrode N. P., or place the sponge-roll N. P. at the soles of the feet, and treat with P. P. upon and a little above the affected parts; using such force of current as the patient can bear. The pain will commonly subside under treatment. If the disease be as low as the ankles or feet, use the *long cord* with N. P.

If the shoulders, arms or hands be affected, treat them on the same principles as are prescribed for the *lower* limbs; using the *long cord* with N. P. when the disease is below the elbows.

When the disease is in the hands or feet, or near to them, if the shoulders or hips be not involved, it is often necessary, after three or four treatments as above described, to *reverse the poles* for a few moments, giving an ascending current; but still using the *long cord* with N. P.

If the disease be located anywhere in the trunk, neck or head, treat the affected part with P. P., placing N. P. on some adjacent part of the spine, and usually at a point somewhat *lower down* than the disease.

For acute inflammatory rheumatism, treat once a day. The length of time for each treatment must depend on the location and extent of the affected part or parts. In this matter, the practitioner must decide for himself, or infer from the time prescribed in the treatment of other inflammatory affections.

RHEUMATISM. (*Chronic.*)

Use the A D current *always* in rheumatic affections. If there be no visible inflammation or swelling in the diseased parts, approach such parts in the same mannėr as in acute inflammatory rheumatism, except with *reversed poles*. The parts affected require to come under the N. P. rather than the P. P., and to be treated with considerable force. There are *apparently* exceptional cases, referred to on page 83, which see.

Where joints are being dislocated, treat the parts with N. P., quite mild force, so long as it can be done without exciting acute inflammation. If this should arise, it must be repressed with P. P.

Treat chronic rheumatism about three times a week.

DROPSY.

Use the A D current, moderate force. Give *general tonic treatment;* then place P. P. with the feet, in a vessel of warm water, or place the sponge-roll P. P. at the soles of the feet, and treat the affected parts a few minutes with N. P., to quicken the absorbents. If the disease be in the feet or lower limbs, use *long cord* with P. P. while treating them. Next place N. P. upon the lower part of the bladder, or, what is better, immediately below the pubic articulation, and treat over the kidneys three to five minutes with P. P. Repeat the treatments about three times a week.

NEURALGIA.

If the disease be general in the system, moving from place to place, or causing transient acute pains here and there, give general tonic treatment, three times a week, for several weeks—perhaps a month or two, provided the case be an old one. This will invigorate the nervous system and equalize the electric action. *Relief* will be afforded soon; but for the sake of *cure*, the treatment of an old case should be continued as here directed. If the disease be *local*, use the B D current, with as much force as the patient can bear without irritating painfulness. Treat the affected part, or parts, with P. P., placing N. P., *long cord*, upon some approximate healthy part, at a point a little lower down than the part in pain. The spine, when convenient, is commonly the best point for it. In treating the painful part, pass the electrode more or less also over the nerves adjacent to the one principally affected. Treat five to eight minutes daily.

SCIATICA.

This is neuralgia in an ischiatic nerve, commonly the *great* ischiatic.

Use the B D current, strong as the patient can well bear. Place the foot in warm water with N. P., or place the sponge-roll N. P. at the sole of the foot, (the former is the best,) and treat with P. P. over the painful part, and also, more or less, over adjacent parts. It is also well, in order to prevent too much exhaustion of the limb, to *reverse the poles* every third or fourth time; but in so doing, use the *long cord* with N. P.

PARALYSIS.

Take the B D current, medium force. If the paralysis be in a lower limb, place P. P., *long cord*, upon the lower lumbar vertebræ, so as to reach the hypogastric plexus, and treat with the metallic brush, N. P., five to eight minutes, over all the affected parts. Then close the sitting with *reversed poles*, about one to two minutes, having P. P., *long cord*, at the foot, and manipulating over the parts affected, and especially over the lumbar vertebræ, with N. P. This is to prevent depletion by *running off* the electro-vital fluid too much, and to force the electric current through the nerves in an upward and inward tonic-giving direction. If the disease be in an arm or hand, treat it in a manner analogous to the above; extending the treatment from back of neck to the affected parts.

In case of *hemiplegia* or *paraplegia*, run the

current from the healthy *side* of the spine, (in hemiplegia,) or from a healthy *part* of the spine, (in paraplegia,) to and through the paralyzed parts, by placing P. P., *long cord*, on spine, and manipulating with N. P., metallic brush commonly, upon the parts paralyzed. Close the treatment with reversed poles for a moment or two, as in the preceding cases. *Old* paralysis requires considerable *time* to cure it. Treat about three times a week, occasionally omitting a week.

ERYSIPELAS.

Take the A. D. current, medium force, in all forms of the diseases.

1. When acute, and characterized by high inflammation, with bright, smooth swelling, and spreading gradually and sometimes rapidly to surrounding parts; or when small vesicles appear on the inflamed parts, which dry up in little branlike scales and fall off.

If it be located anywhere upon the face, place N. P., *long cord*, upon back of neck, and treat the parts affected with P. P. Treat about three to five minutes at a time, three or four times daily.

If it be located in the arm or hand, place

the extremity in tepid water with N. P., *long cord*, and treat upon or just above the diseased part with P. P.

If it be in any part of the trunk, (which, in this form, is not so common,) place N. P., *long cord*, upon some point of the spine as near the diseased part as may be, but a little lower down, and treat the part affected with P. P.

In each of these cases, treat briefly, but frequently, as directed above.

2. When small, blister-like, serous vesicles—*phlyctæna*—appear, and the inflammation terminates in gangrene; or when there is such an infiltration of serum as to produce an œdemetous condition, place P. P., *long cord*, upon some convenient healthy part, (the spinal cord, or other nerve centre which gives nervous service to the part affected, is best,) and treat the lesion with N. P., *light force*, five to eight minutes daily.

ERUPTIVE CUTANEOUS DISEASES.

Take A D current, pretty *vigorous* force in *acute* cases; *mild* in *chronic* affections. If the eruption be inflamed and acute, use *long cord* with N. P.; if sluggish and chronic, use *long cord* with P. P. Move the two electrodes parallel to each other, upon the patient, about two or three inches apart; and pass them over all the affected surface. Repeat the treatment daily in acute affections, and three times a week in chronic cases.

COMMON CRAMP.

Although either the positive or the negative pole, applied to the healthy muscle, may produce spasmodic contraction, yet the negative pole contracts much more powerfully than the positive—a fact which shows an electrically *plus* condition in the nerves and muscles involved. Yet we know that cramps are more apt to attend a *low* condition of general vitality in the system than the opposite. From several considerations, which can not be detailed here, I am led to think that cramps are produced, generally, at least, by a temporary or spasmodic *reaction* of the electro-vital force from an improperly negative to an excessively positive state in the parts affected.

My practice is, when the spasm is on, to treat the parts in cramp by momentary touches rapidly repeated, with the P. P. of the B D or A D current, good medium force, placing N. P. at the back of neck, if the disturbance be in an arm; or at the coccyx, if it be in a leg or in the abdomen or chest.

In treating parts subject to cramp while the spasm is *not* on, give them, along with other parts of the system, *general tonic treatment*, as directed on page 95. This elevates and equalizes the electro-vital action, and relieves the difficulty.

TRISMUS. (*Lockjaw.*)

For traumatic trismus, use the B D current, of vigorous force. Let the wound be kept open and clear, except that soothing emollients may be applied. Place N. P. at the coccyx, or near it on the spine; and then treat, by firm but momentary touches of the P. P., over the lower maxillary—*pterygoid*—muscles and nerves; indeed, over the *entire* lower jaw and its articulations. Treat five to ten minutes, if necessary, or until the jaws relax.

TETANUS.

This is substantially the same thing as *trismus*, except that it extends to other parts, and often to nearly all the muscles of the organism. Under ordinary treatment, it is almost invariably fatal. I am not aware that it has been sufficiently submitted to *our* electrical system to determine satisfactorily the question of its amenability to it. Yet I see no reason to doubt that, in the most of cases, when taken within reasonable time, it may be cured.

Use the B D current, in pretty strong force. Place the N. P., *long cord*, at the feet, and treat with P. P. from the medulla oblongata, or from the upper cervical vertebra, all along down the spine, for several minutes—say, three to five minutes. Then pass with P. P. over the whole trunk and limbs. Continue to treat until relaxation takes place, or all hope of relief departs.

CANCERS.

Cancers take on a variety of forms, distinguished by different names; but since they all require substantially the same electrical treatment, it is unnecessary here to describe them.

Begin with the A B current in pretty full volume. [The *volume* of the current is increased by increasing the quantity of battery fluid.] Use this for several weeks, and then change to the A D current. Treat daily. The time for each treatment must be determined by the judgment of the practitioner; varying it according to the peculiar character and location of the disease.

If the cancer be on the face, or on any part of the head or breast, place P. P. on back of neck; but if it be in the stomach, uterus, or any of the abdominal viscera, place P. P. on spine, a little higher than the affected part. Then treat the disease with N. P., *long cord*, so as to run the current immediately *out* from the lesion, and yet bring the latter on the *negative* side * of the central point in the circuit; that is, within the negative half of the whole circuit.

ASPHYXIA. (*Suspended Animation.*)

Use B D current, pretty strong force. Place P. P. at back of neck—second or third cervical vertebra, and treat with N. P., over all the chest and along the lower margin of the ribs, so as to excite the pectoral muscles, lungs and diaphragm.

---

* See *Polarization of the Circuit.* Page 29.

RECENT WOUNDS, CONTUSIONS AND BURNS.

Use the B D current, strong force as can be borne. Bring the lesion under P. P., and place N. P. at discretion, in view of the location of the injury. Treat five to eight minutes, twice or thrice on the same day. Unless the injury is very severe, no further treatment will be required. Healing will take place with little or no soreness or swelling. In severe cases, repeat the treatment whenever inflammation gets too high. If *fungus*—"proud flesh"—should appear, treat that with a small-pointed electrode, N. P., placing P. P. on a healthy part, not remote, using A C current, in pretty strong force.

OLD ULCERS.

Take the A D current. If *torpid*, treat with mild force. Treat the sore with N. P., while P. P. is held upon some healthy part, and usually at a higher point. Treat five to ten minutes, three or four times a week. If *high inflammation* be present, this must first be reduced by applying P. P., in pretty strong force, with N. P., on a healthy part not far away. For this purpose, treat some five to eight minutes daily. Then, when the inflammation is sufficiently subdued, treat as when *torpid*, with mild force and less frequently. It is best, when it can be done, to place the affected part in warm water along with N. P.; bringing the ulcer immediately above the surface of the water.

HEMORRHAGE.

Take B D current, strong force. Apply P. P. to the open blood-vessel, or as near to it as possible; placing N. P., *long cord*, to some adjacent part, and, as nearly as practicable, in the direction from which the blood chiefly comes.

CHLOROSIS. (*Green Sickness.*)

This is a disease mostly or entirely peculiar to young women who have not menstruated, and disappears on the establishment of the monthly periods.

Take the A D current. If any symptoms exist of an effort of nature to bring on the menses, note the *time* of them, and regard it, in the treatment, as the proper monthly period. If no symptoms of such a period are perceptible, the practitioner must *fix* upon a time for it, and regard it accordingly. About four to six days before the periodic time, commence to treat as follows, using a *moderate force:* Insert the uterine electrode, N. P., wet in warm water, per vagina, until it meets the uterus; and manipulate with P. P. over the dorsal and first two lumbar vertebræ, and more or less over the back on both sides of the spinal column, some six or eight minutes daily, down to the period fixed upon for the catamenia to appear. If they do not start, let the patient rest for some four or five days, and then begin with *general tonic treatment.* (See page 95.) Continue this, three times a week, until within a little less than a week of the *periodic* time, when the same treatment with the uterine electrode as was at first employed should be resumed, and again be continued to the time assigned for the menses. If no success should appear, return, after a few days, to *general tonic treatment* as before. Let these forms of treatment be prosecuted until success crowns the effort. Ordinarily, not many months—perhaps not more than one or two months—will be required; especially, if the treatment be aided, on the part of the patient, by a good degree of moderate exercise in the open air, and a free, nourishing diet.

AMENORRHŒA. (*Suppressed Menstruation.*)

Treat as for *chlorosis.* But if the case be recent—the effect of taking cold—begin, in the first few sittings, to treat eight or ten minutes as for common cold; then conclude the sitting by treating, about as many minutes, in the same manner as prescribed for chlorosis.

DYSMENORRHŒA. (*Painful Menstruation.*)

If the disease be occasioned by uterine displacement, obstructing the *os uteri,* the organ must be restored to its normal position. This can best be done by mechanical action. But it is most commonly occasioned by irritation of the mucus membrane lining the interior cavity of the uterus. Mucus surfaces, under *chronic* irritation, are electrically negative. Therefore, in this case, if it be an *old* one, taking the A D current, *very mild force,* apply the uterine electrode, N. P., to the *os uteri,* and treat over the lower dorsal and upper lumbar vertebræ with P. P., *long cord.* Treat five to eight minutes, three times a week.

But I should add, that recovery from this infirmity, when occasioned by uterine irritation, will be much aided by commencing each sitting with a *general tonic treatment* (see page 95), and closing with the treatment just above prescribed.

The last described form of dysmenorrhœa is sometimes attended with spasmodic contraction of the *os uteri*, thus preventing the catamenial flow. This may be readily relieved by applying P. P. to uterus, and N. P. to lower dorsal and upper lumbar vertebræ.

MENORRHAGIA. (*Excessive Menstruation.*)

If the menstrual flow is apt to terminate in hemorrhage, it is best to give *general tonic treatments*, about three times a week, between the periods; and during the last four or five days before color is expected to appear, to take the B D current, medium force, and treat the uterus directly, once a day, with the uterine electrode P. P., while moving N. P. over the dorsal vertebræ, about five to eight minutes, at the close of *general tonic treatment.*

If there be no *hemorrhage*, properly, but only too profuse or too long-continued flow of catamenia, the discharge may commonly be stopped by one or two treatments, of eight to ten minutes each, with the uterine electrode, as prescribed above.

PROLAPSUS UTERI. (*Falling of the Womb.*)

Take the B D current, of good medium force, and give *general tonic treatment* (see page 95), on alternate days, ten minutes, passing briefly over the several parts. After this, treat five to eight minutes with uterine electrode, in the manner prescribed for *menorrhagia.* Then close the sitting by removing the uterine instrument, substituting the sponge-cup as P. P., and treating with it externally, about five minutes, over the pelvic region, while N. P. is stationed on the spine, at the first or second dorsal vertebra.

On the *intervening* days, treat only with the uterine electrode, as above prescribed.

LEUCORRHŒA. (*Whites.*)

Take A D current, *very mild* force. Introduce the vaginal electrode, N. P., until it meets the uterus, and manipulate with P. P. over the dorsal vertebræ five to eight minutes, three times a week. Once or twice a week, on the intervening days, give *general tonic treatment.* Omit treatment altogether, for one or two weeks, once in two to three months.

Considerable time is often required for the cure of old cases.

SPERMATORRHŒA.

The points to be gained are, to reduce the action of the amatorial organs of the brain and the secretion of the *testes*, and to contract and strengthen the tissue of the seminal vesicles and the prostrate gland.

Take the B D current. First, treat the lowest part of the cerebellum, on both sides of the spinal cord, with a *mild* force; using P. P. upon these organs of amativeness, and N. P. on the dorsal vertebræ. Treat so some three minutes. Next, increase the current to medium force; and, taking a handled cup or mug, holding a pint to a quart, mostly filled with tepid water, drop the *penis* and *testicles* into it, along with the tin electrode P. P., and move N. P., *long cord*, over the lumbar vertebræ. Treat in this manner about five minutes. Then place the P. P. on the pelvis, close above the penis, and again treat with N. P., *long cord*, over the small of the back, two or three minutes. Treat about three times a week.

IMPOTENCE.

Take B D current, moderate force. Treat exactly as in spermatorrhœa, except with *reversed poles*, using the *long cord* with P. P. Treat thrice a week.

www.ingramcontent.com/pod-product-compliance
Lightning Source LLC
LaVergne TN
LVHW021410110826
845150LV00007B/1863

* 9 7 8 1 4 2 5 5 1 1 1 1 1 *